This book is due for return on or before the last date shown below.

Colour Atlas of
Ophthalmic
Plastic Surgery

To Renée, Jonathan, Richard, Johanna and Rebecca

For Churchill Livingstone
Commissioning Editor: Michael Parkinson
Project Editor: Dilys Jones
Copy Editor: Pat Croucher
Design Direction: Sarah Cape
Paste-up Artist: Jim Farley
Project Controller: Nancy Arnott
Sales Promotion Executive: Douglas McNaughton

Colour Atlas of Ophthalmic Plastic Surgery

A. G. Tyers
FRCS (Eng) FRCS (Ed) FRCOphth
Consultant Ophthalmic Surgeon,
Odstock Hospital,
Salisbury

J. R. O. Collin
MA FRCS FRCOphth
Consultant Ophthalmic Surgeon,
Moorfields Eye Hospital and the Institute of Ophthalmology,
University of London

Illustrations by Terry R. Tarrant
FMAA

Churchill Livingstone

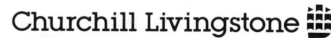

EDINBURGH HONG KONG LONDON MADRID MELBOURNE NEW YORK AND TOKYO 1995

CHURCHILL LIVINGSTONE
Medical Division of Longman Group Limited

Distributed in the United States of America by Churchill Livingstone
Inc., 650 Avenue of the Americas, New York, N. Y. 10011, and by
associated companies, branches and representatives throughout the
world.

First published 1995

ISBN 0-443-04452-X

British Library Cataloguing in Publication Data
A catalogue record for this book is available from the British Library.

Library of Congress Cataloging in Publication Data
A catalog record for this book is available from the Library of
Congress.

The
publisher's
policy is to use
**paper manufactured
from sustainable forests**

Printed in Hong Kong
GC/01

Contents

Acknowledgements

We are very grateful to the Department of Medical Photography in Salisbury, especially to Richard Bolton and Stephen Moore who took most of the surgical photographs. They often made themselves available at short notice and their enthusiasm was a great asset to the project. We would also like to thank David Candish, in charge of the ophthalmic operating theatre in Salisbury, whose planning and experience allowed the surgery and photography to proceed as smoothly as possible. Our thanks also extend to Bob McDowall, consultant plastic surgeon in Salisbury in the Regional Unit for Plastic and Reconstructive Surgery, who made valuable comments on those parts of the atlas which overlap with general plastic surgery. Finally, we would like to record our debt to the many colleagues and friends who have encouraged us over the years. Of the many we could name we are especially grateful to Dr Charles Beyer-Machule and Dr Crowell Beard who encouraged us as we embarked on our careers in ophthalmic plastic surgery and who have remained our valued mentors and friends ever since.

CHAPTER 1

Anatomy

The eyelids protect the eyes. Disease which alters eyelid structure or function threatens sight and an understanding of eyelid anatomy and physiology is fundamental to good reconstructive surgery. The eyelids should not be studied in isolation but in the context of the surrounding structures.

1.1 The bony orbit
(Diags 1.1,2)

The orbits are roughly pyramidal spaces with parallel medial walls. In cross-section they are rectangular anteriorly and triangular posteriorly. Each orbit is about 4 cm deep and has a volume of about 30 ml. The apex is the optic foramen which is separated from the superior orbital fissure laterally by a thin bar of bone. The inferior orbital fissure extends interiorly and laterally from just below the optic foramen; about midway along its length the infraorbital groove branches anteriorly.

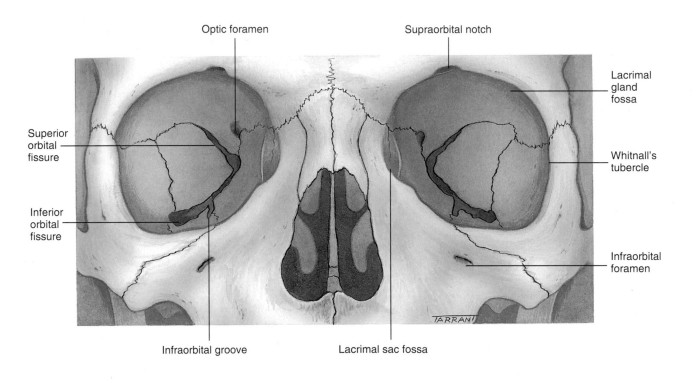

Optic foramen

Supraorbital notch

Lacrimal gland fossa

Superior orbital fissure

Whitnall's tubercle

Inferior orbital fissure

Infraorbital foramen

Infraorbital groove

Lacrimal sac fossa

Diag. 1.1

The lateral orbital walls are at 45 degrees to the medial walls and 90 degrees to each other. The floor, narrow at the apex, broadens as it slopes down and laterally. It is separated from the lateral wall by the inferior orbital fissure and it is continuous with the medial wall. The junction of the medial wall and the roof is marked by the anterior and posterior ethmoidal foramina about 3–4 cm from the orbital rim.

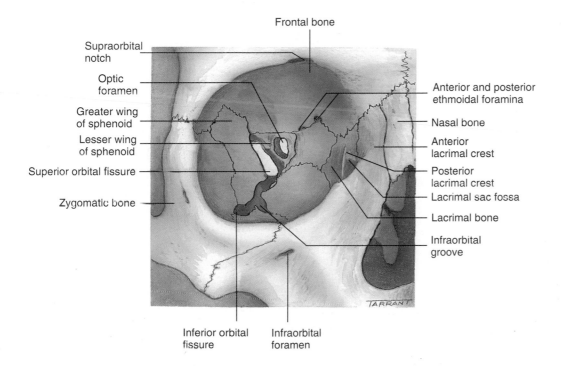

Diag. 1.2

The fossa for the lacrimal gland is just posterior to the superolateral orbital rim. The lacrimal sac fossa is just posterior to the inferomedial orbital rim, bounded anteriorly by the anterior lacrimal crest, a continuation of the inferior orbital rim, and posteriorly by the posterior lacrimal crest, a continuation of the superior orbital rim.

Each orbital margin measures approximately 40 mm although the horizontal margins are usually greater than the vertical. The lateral rim is posterior to the medial rim and this is more marked in children. Just within the mid-point of the lateral rim Whitnall's (lateral orbital) tubercle may be palpated. The trochlea is palpable just within the superomedial rim. The supraorbital notch is at the junction of the medial third and the lateral two-thirds of the superior rim and the infraorbital foramen is about 5 mm below the mid-point of the inferior rim or just medial to this.

The orbits are lined by periosteum (periorbita) which can be lifted easily (see Figs 12.3c, 13.7c) except at the orbital margins, at the sutures, fissures and foramina, and at the margins of the lacrimal sac fossa. At the posterior lacrimal crest the periosteum splits to enclose the lacrimal sac and reunites at the anterior lacrimal crest.

The orbits are a protection and support for the eyes and they transmit nerves and vessels to the face.

1.2 Surface anatomy of the eyelids *(Figs 1.1–1.4)*

The upper and lower lids enclose the palpebral aperture and they join at the medial and lateral canthi. The average size of the palpebral aperture in an adult is 30 mm horizontally and 10 mm vertically between the centres of the lids. The point of maximum concavity is different in the two lids. In the upper lid it is medial to the pupil, in the lower lid it is lateral. With the eye in the primary position the upper lid covers 1–3 mm of the upper cornea and the lower lid is at or close to the lower limbus.

In the upper lid the delicate preseptal skin (inferior to the brow) and the pretarsal skin (superior to the lashes) meet at the level of the skin crease – 6–10 mm from the lash line in an adult, lower in a child. The skin crease is formed by the insertion of the levator aponeurosis into the orbicularis muscle at this level – usually approximately at the superior border of the tarsal plate (Diag. 1.6). There is often redundant skin superior to the skin crease in the upper lid so that a skin fold is created which covers the skin crease (Fig. 1.1). Superior to the skin crease the 'fullness' in the upper lid (Fig. 1.2) is due to orbital fat. The lacrimal gland lies laterally. Immediately below the brow there may be some hollowing of the upper lid – the upper lid sulcus (see Fig. 1.1). This is often marked in the elderly, especially if there is a ptosis (see Fig. 9.2 Pre).

If a skin crease is present in the lower lid it is usually less obvious than the upper lid crease which is more frequently double. It is formed approximately at the level of the lower border of the inferior tarsal plate, 4–5 mm from the lash line (Diag 1.8).

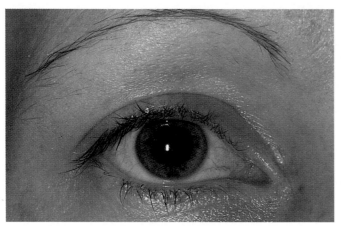

Fig. 1.1

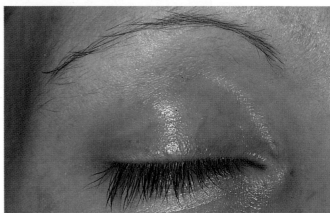

Fig. 1.2

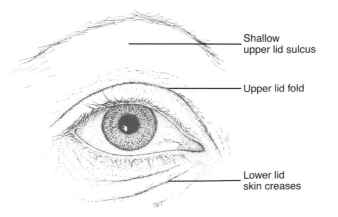

Shallow
upper lid sulcus

Upper lid fold

Lower lid
skin creases

Key diag. 1.1

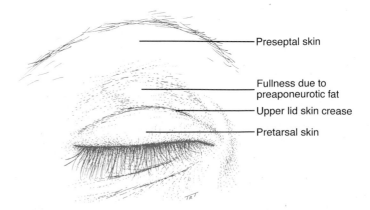

Preseptal skin

Fullness due to
preaponeurotic fat

Upper lid skin crease

Pretarsal skin

Key diag. 1.2

The brow lies along the anterior aspect of the superior orbital rim. As the orbital rim descends laterally the downward curve of the brow is more gentle. In contrast to the thin skin of the upper lid, brow skin is thick (see Fig. 10.7e). It bears numerous hairs whose follicles are directed laterally at about 30 degrees, except at the medial end of the brow where they are directed upwards.

In upgaze the action of the levator and Muller's muscles lifts the upper eyelid. The action of the frontalis lifts the brow. The elevation of the brow contributes about 2 mm to the elevation of the upper lid. The lateral canthus rises slightly. The upper lid fold is accentuated.

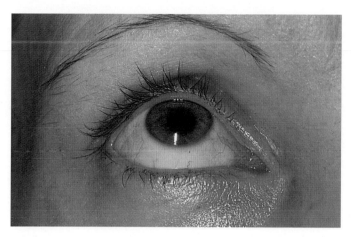

Fig. 1.3

In downgaze the lower lid level is depressed by the pull of the lower lid retractors and the lower lid skin crease is accentuated. The lateral canthus moves down slightly. The upper lid fold is reduced revealing the previously covered skin crease.

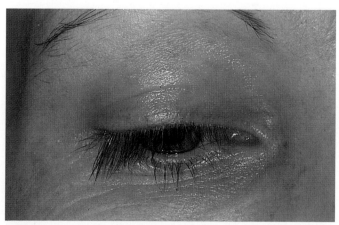

Fig. 1.4

1.3 Eyelid structure

The eyelids are conveniently divided into two anatomical lamellae (Diags 1.6, 1.8). The anterior lid lamella includes the skin and the orbicularis muscle. The posterior lamella is formed by the tarsal plate and the conjunctiva. These lamellae are very important in eyelid surgery. Between the layers of the lamellae there are connective tissue layers.

The margins of the eyelids are 2 mm wide. The posterior lid margin is sharp and applied to the globe, the anterior lid margin is rounded and holds the eyelashes. A grey line, visible along the middle of each lid margin, marks the junction of the anterior and posterior lamellae of the lid (see Fig. 3.12b). The openings of the Meibomian glands are just posterior to this line.

The layers of the eyelids will now be discussed in more detail.

1.4 Eyelid skin

The skin of the eyelids is the thinnest in the body, less than 1 mm thick and almost transparent in places (see Fig. 9.4a). It is attached quite loosely to the orbicularis muscle and more firmly to the region of the canthal tendons – especially the medial. The mucocutaneous junction is at the Meibomian gland openings.

Apart from the lashes the skin hairs are very fine. Sweat glands of Moll secrete between the lashes or into the ducts of the glands of Zeis. The sebaceous glands of Zeis secrete into the lash follicles.

Deep to the skin is a thin layer of loose connective tissue which contains no fat and which lies on the orbicularis muscle.

1.5 The striated muscle layer and canthal tendons *(Diags 1.3–1.5)*

The orbicularis oculi muscle is the main protractor of the eyelids. The muscle is a flat sheet of fibres which encircles the palpebral aperture spreading out beyond the orbital rim. It is divided into concentric zones – orbital and palpebral. The palpebral part is divided into preseptal and pretarsal parts.

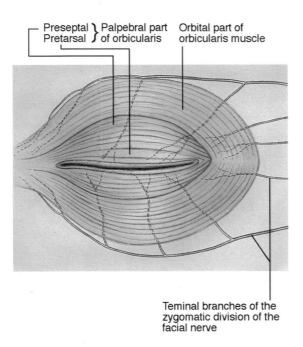

Preseptal ⎱ Palpebral part   Orbital part of
Pretarsal ⎰ of orbicularis   orbicularis muscle

Teminal branches of the zygomatic division of the facial nerve

Diag. 1.3

The orbital part lies over and beyond the orbital rim. It arises from the superior and inferior medial orbital rim and its fibres sweep laterally in concentric bands to join at the lateral orbital rim. The palpebral parts insert medially and arise from the lateral canthal tendon. The preseptal part lies anterior to the orbital septum in the upper and lower lids and the pretarsal part lies on the tarsal plates. At the lid margins the pretarsal muscle extends posteriorly as far as the Meibomian gland openings as the muscle of Riolan (Diags 1.6, 1.8).

1.5a The lateral canthal tendon

The pretarsal muscles join laterally and insert by a common tendon into Whitnall's tubercle. The preseptal muscles join laterally to form a lateral raphe which is connected to the underlying tendon. Deep to the muscle insertions a Y-shaped fibrous thickening in the orbital septum joins the lateral ends of the tarsal plates to Whitnall's tubercle. These structures together form the lateral canthal tendon.

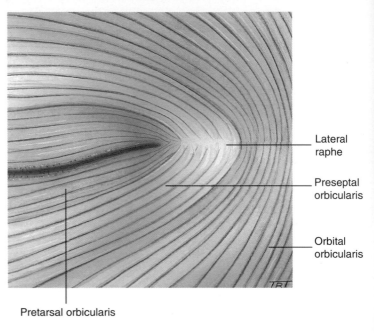

Lateral raphe

Preseptal orbicularis

Orbital orbicularis

Pretarsal orbicularis

Diag. 1.4

1.5b *The medial canthal tendon*

The medial canthal tendon also has a fibrous and a muscular component.

The fibrous component is attached laterally to the medial ends of the tarsal plates as two limbs of a Y and it inserts medially on the frontal process of the maxilla just anterior to the anterior lacrimal crest, level with the upper part of the lacrimal sac. It has a definite inferior border but the superior border blends with the periosteum. A posterior part leaves the deep surface just lateral to the anterior lacrimal crest and inserts into the posterior lacrimal crest behind the lacrimal sac.

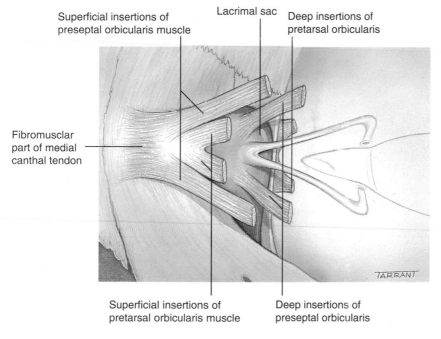

Superficial insertions of preseptal orbicularis muscle

Lacrimal sac

Deep insertions of pretarsal orbicularis

Fibromusclar part of medial canthal tendon

Superficial insertions of pretarsal orbicularis muscle

Deep insertions of preseptal orbicularis

Dlag. 1.5

The pretarsal muscles, firmly attached to the tarsal plates, insert medially by a superficial head and a deep head. The superficial head from each lid blends with the fibrous component to form the anterior part of the medial canthal tendon. The deep head from each lid is also known as the pars lacrimalis, or Horner's muscle. Its fibres begin at the medial ends of the tarsal plates and insert into the posterior lacrimal crest a few millimetres behind the lacrimal sac. Contraction of the deep head pulls the lid medially and posteriorly.

The preseptal muscles, less firmly attached to the orbital septum, also insert medially by a superficial and a deep head. The superficial head from each lid inserts into the superficial part of the medial canthal tendon. The deep heads insert into the fascia overlying the lacrimal sac and on the medial orbital wall above and below Horner's muscle. Contraction of the deep heads pulls the lacrimal fascia laterally.

There is some discussion about the detailed anatomy of the medial canthus. In practice the individual muscle insertions described above are not usually identified at operation.

1.5c The lacrimal pump

During blinking the deep heads of the pretarsal muscles (Horner's muscle) pull the medial ends of the eyelids medially, shortening the canaliculi, while the lacrimal fascia and sac wall are pulled laterally by contraction of the deep heads of the preseptal muscle. The puncta close and tears in the ampullae of the canaliculi are forced medially and are sucked into the sac. As the deep insertions of the orbicularis muscle relax at the end of the blink the lacrimal fascia and sac wall move medially again, the medial ends of the lids move laterally, the puncta reopen and the ampullae refill with tears. Drainage of tears from the lacrimal sac into the nasolacrimal duct is not due to the lacrimal pump mechanism and is mainly due to gravity.

1.5d Corrugator supercilii muscle

This small muscle arises from the medial end of the superciliary ridge and passes upwards and laterally through both frontalis and orbicularis to insert into the skin of the middle of the brow.

1.5e Procerus muscle

This small muscle arises on the nasal bones and inserts into the skin of the lower forehead and bridge of the nose.

1.5f Occipitofrontalis muscle

Occipitalis muscle posteriorly and frontalis muscle anteriorly are joined by an aponeurosis, the galea aponeurotica or epicranial aponeurosis. Laterally it blends with the temporalis fascia. The frontalis muscle fibres insert into the orbicularis muscle and the skin of the brows. The galea splits to enclose the frontalis muscle. The anterior part covers the anterior surface of the orbicularis muscle. The posterior part splits again to enclose the fat pad of the brow. The anterior layer covers the posterior surface of orbicularis and the posterior layer becomes the orbital septum.

1.6 The retro-orbicular fascia and related spaces

Posterior to the orbicularis muscle is areolar tissue containing the vessels and nerves of the lids and a variable amount of fat. Dissection in this space splits a lid into its two lamellae (e.g. see Fig. 8.2b).

In the lower lid (Diag. 1.8) the relations of this space are the orbicularis anteriorly and the tarsal plate and septum posteriorly (see Figs 10.6b, 18.5b).

In the upper lid (Diag. 1.6) the equivalent space posterior to the orbicularis muscle is subdivided by the levator aponeurosis which passes between the inferior border of the septum and the superior border of the tarsal plate to insert into the orbicularis muscle and the anterior surface of the tarsal plate (see Fig 9.4b). A well defined surgical space can be identified posterior to the aponeurosis – the postaponeurotic space (see Fig. 9.4f). It is limited anteriorly by the aponeurosis, posteriorly by the tarsal plate below and Muller's muscle above, superiorly by the attachment of Muller's muscle to the levator and inferiorly by the attachment of the aponeurosis to the lower anterior surface of the tarsal plate. When the upper lid is in the anatomical position this space is shallow and Muller's muscle lies in close approximation to the levator aponeurosis. However, if the lid is everted the space changes shape separating the lower ends of the two upper lid retractors (Diag. 1.7). A less well defined, potential space is present anterior to the aponeurosis (see Figs 9.4a, b). It is limited anteriorly by the orbicularis muscle, posteriorly by the septum above and the anterior surface of the aponeurosis below, inferiorly by the lid margin and superiorly by the preseptal fat extending inferiorly from beneath the brow. This space is interrupted at the level of the skin crease by the insertion of the aponeurosis into the orbicularis muscle. In ptosis surgery from the anterior approach it is important that the dissection upwards to expose the septum remains in this space, immediately posterior to the orbicularis, and does not stray into the space posterior to the aponeurosis where the dissection is deceptively easier (see Figs 9.2b,c, 9.4f).

1.7 The septum and tarsal plates

The junction of the periorbita and the periosteum at the orbital rim is thickened to form the arcus marginalis and from this the septum passes into the lids. In each lid the septum does not reach the proximal border of the tarsal plate but fuses with the upper or lower lid retractors 2–4 mm from the tarsus (see Diags 1.6, 1.8, Fig. 9.4b).

The origin of the septum crosses the supraorbital notch, descends the lateral orbital wall to enclose the structures inserted into Whitnall's tubercle then descends to the inferotemporal angle of the orbit. Here the origin passes just anterior to the rim then turns medially across the inferior orbital rim to the lower part of the anterior lacrimal crest. It passes posteriorly attached to the lacrimal fascia approximately at the middle of the sac to reach to the posterior lacrimal crest. It encloses the deep heads of the orbicularis and ascends the posterior lacrimal crest to the superomedial angle of the orbit where it turns laterally onto the superior rim.

The septum is related to the orbicularis muscle anteriorly and the orbital fat posteriorly (see Diags 1.6, 1.8. Figs 10.1e,f, 10.2a). It is pierced by vessels and nerves and by the insertion of the levator aponeurosis into the orbicularis at the level of the upper tarsal border.

The tarsal plates form the skeleton of the eyelids. They are made of dense fibrous tissue with some elastic tissue. The Meibomian glands lie within the substance of the tarsal plates. The vessels and nerves of the lids lie on their anterior surfaces within loose connective tissue. In the upper lid the lower fibres of the levator aponeurosis insert into the lower part of the tarsal plate and Muller's muscle is attached to the proximal border (see Fig. 9.2e). In the lower lid the lower lid retractors insert into the proximal border (see Fig. 6.4c). The tarsal conjunctiva is firmly attached to their posterior surfaces.

1.8 The conjunctiva

Mucus-secreting goblet cells are plentiful everywhere in the conjunctiva. The accessory lacrimal glands of Wolfring and Krause are found mainly between the upper tarsal border and the upper fornix especially laterally (Diag. 1.6). The lacrimal gland ducts empty into the lateral part of the upper fornix.

The superior and inferior fornices extend almost to the orbital rims. The lateral fornix extends to approximately 14 mm from the limbus but the medial fornix is shallower. Fibrous tissue support reaches the fornices and in the superior and inferior fornices 'suspensory ligaments' can be identified (Diags 1.6, 1.8). They are extensions of the common sheaths between the upper or lower lid retractors and the superior or inferior rectus muscles.

1.9 The upper lid retractors *(Diag. 1.6)*

The normal position of the upper lid is maintained by the levator and Muller's muscles working together.

The levator muscle arises from the roof of the orbit immediately in front of the optic foramen and above the superior rectus muscle (Diag. 1.14). It passes forwards (see Figs 9.7b,c) for about 40 mm where it ends just behind the septum as an aponeurosis (see Figs 9.4d, 9.5c). Close to the origin of the aponeurosis the muscle sheath is thickened above the muscle to form a band, Whitnall's ligament (Diags 1.6, 1.9). This may be a definite structure, easily seen, or a more diffuse thickening (see Figs 9.4d,k,l, 9.5c). It inserts into the trochlea medially and the capsule of the lacrimal gland and orbital wall laterally. It acts as a fulcrum for the action of the levator.

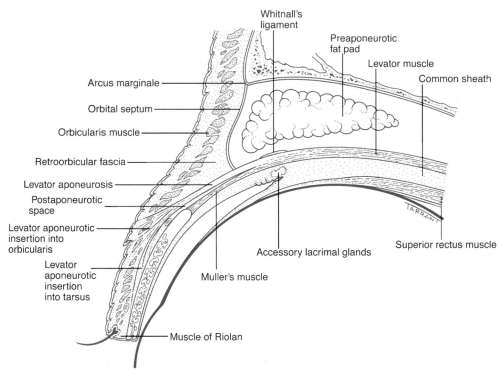

Diag. 1.6

The levator aponeurosis descends into the lid and the septum inserts onto its anterior surface, often as a thickened band, about 8 mm below Whitnall's ligament and 3–4 mm above the tarsus (see Figs 9.4b, 9.5a). The angle between the posterior surface of the septum and the levator muscle contains the preaponeurotic fat pad – an important surgical landmark (see Figs 9.2d, 9.4c). As the aponeurosis descends it becomes thinner and fans out. It inserts anteriorly into the orbicularis muscle at the level of the skin crease and below, into the lower anterior surface of the tarsal plate. Its lateral insertion is as two 'horns' into the region of the canthal tendons (see Diag. 1.9, Figs 9.4f,g, 9.5d). The lacrimal gland is wrapped around the posterior edge of the lateral horn. An extension of the common muscle sheath between the levator and the superior rectus muscle inserts into the superior fornix as the superior suspensory ligament of the fornix.

Muller's smooth muscle arises from the undersurface of the levator muscle (see Figs 9.3c, 11.1c,d) close to the junction of striated muscle and aponeurosis. It is 15–20 mm wide and it descends between the levator aponeurosis and the conjunctiva for about 15–20 mm to insert into the upper border of the tarsal plate (see Figs 9.4f, 10.3c). Note that the lower ends of Muller's muscle and the levator aponeurosis are separated if the upper lid is inverted.

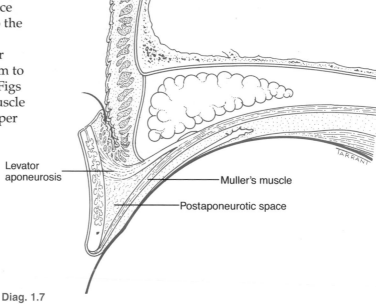

Levator aponeurosis — Muller's muscle — Postaponeurotic space

Diag. 1.7

1.10 *The lower lid retractors* (*Diag. 1.8*)

The developmental capsulopalpebral head of the inferior rectus muscle is the vestigial equivalent of the upper lid retractors and it becomes the lower lid retractors. It arises from the sheath of the inferior rectus muscle and consists of the capsulopalpebral fascia (the levator) and the inferior tarsal muscle (Muller's muscle). It is mainly fibrous tissue but it does contain a small amount of smooth muscle.

As it passes forwards it splits to enclose the inferior oblique muscle and where it reunites it blends with thickened fascia on its inferior aspect. This is Lockwood's suspensory ligament which inserts into the orbital walls close to the canthal tendons. The septum fuses with the lower lid retractors about 2–3 mm below their insertion into the lower tarsal border (see Figs 6.2c, 6.4c, 11.7b, c, 18.5b). The angle between the posterior aspect of the septum and the lower lid retractors contains a pad of orbital fat similar to the preaponeurotic fat in the upper lid (see Fig. 6.4b).

The pull of the lower lid retractors depresses the lid in downgaze and helps to maintain the upright position of the tarsal plate.

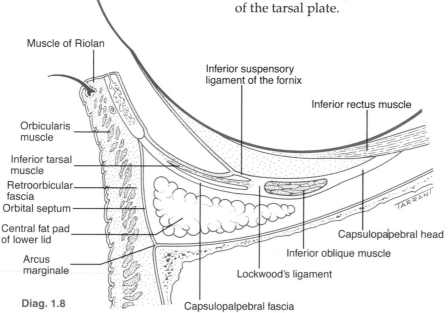

Muscle of Riolan
Inferior suspensory ligament of the fornix
Inferior rectus muscle
Orbicularis muscle
Inferior tarsal muscle
Retroorbicular fascia
Orbital septum
Central fat pad of lower lid
Arcus marginale
Capsulopalpebral head
Inferior oblique muscle
Lockwood's ligament
Capsulopalpebral fascia

Diag. 1.8

1.11 Orbital fat

The muscle cone divides the orbital fat into two parts, intraconal and extraconal fat, which are separated anteriorly but communicate posteriorly. The fat is supported by a complex meshwork of delicate connective tissue septa. The intraconal fat is exposed by enucleation or surgery in the intraconal space. The extraconal fat is frequently seen in lid surgery and is divided into four lobes or fat pads (Diag. 1.9).

In the upper lid there are two fat pads, a smaller medial fat pad and a larger lateral, or central, fat pad, the preaponeurotic fat pad, (see Figs 9.4b,c, 10.3a,b) separated by a fascial septum in the region of the trochlea. Lateral to the preaponeurotic fat pad lies the lacrimal gland.

1.12 The lacrimal gland

The lacrimal gland is wrapped around the posterior border of the lateral horn of the levator aponeurosis (Diags 1.9, 1.14). The superior, orbital part of the gland lies in the lacrimal fossa. Anteriorly it is in contact with the septum and posteriorly with orbital fat. Inferiorly the lateral rectus muscle lies laterally and the levator lies medially. Its secretory ducts pass down into the inferior, palpebral part of the gland which is one-third the size of the orbital part. The anterior border of the palpebral part can be seen laterally in the upper fornix and its secretory ducts emerge there.

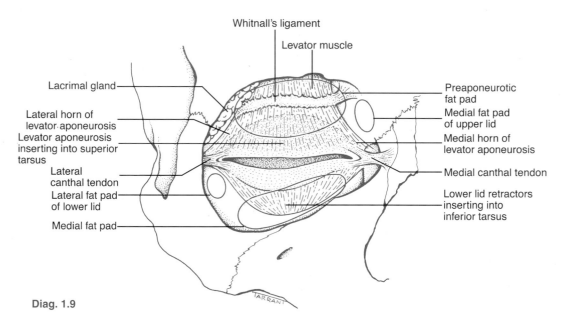

Whitnall's ligament

Levator muscle

Lacrimal gland

Lateral horn of
levator aponeurosis

Levator aponeurosis
inserting into superior
tarsus

Lateral
canthal tendon

Lateral fat pad
of lower lid

Medial fat pad

Preaponeurotic
fat pad

Medial fat pad
of upper lid

Medial horn of
levator aponeurosis

Medial canthal tendon

Lower lid retractors
inserting into
inferior tarsus

Diag. 1.9

In the lower lid there are also two fat pads (see Figs 6.4b, 10.6b, c, 18.5b). The larger medial fat pad is often subdivided into two smaller collections by a septum in the region of the inferior oblique muscle origin. The smaller lateral fat pad is separated from the medial fat pad(s) by a fascial septum.

1.13 The lacrimal sac

The lacrimal canaliculi, surrounded by orbicularis muscle immediately medial to the puncta, pass medially and posteriorly between the limbs of the medial canthal tendon to reach its posterior aspect and there pierce the fascia overlying the lacrimal sac. They usually join to form a common canaliculus before entering the sac (Diag. 1.5).

The sac lies in the lacrimal (sac) fossa. Periosteum at the posterior lacrimal crest splits to enclose the sac and reunites at the anterior lacrimal crest. The lateral leaf is the stronger and it is reinforced further by the posterior leaf of the medial canthal tendon. The anterior part of the tendon crosses the upper part of the sac and the septum covers the lower part. The inferior oblique muscle arises just behind and lateral to the orifice of the nasolacrimal duct. Anterior to the medial canthal tendon, 8 mm medial to the medial canthus, is the angular vein.

1.14 Blood supply to the lids *(Diags 1.10, 1.11)*

1.14a Arterial supply

The ophthalmic artery gives origin to the lacrimal artery lateral to the optic nerve and to the supraorbital artery as it crosses the optic nerve to reach the medial wall. It terminates by dividing into the dorsal nasal and supratrochlear arteries. Other branches supply the orbit.

The lacrimal artery passes forward on the upper border of the lateral rectus muscle accompanied by the lacrimal nerve. It supplies the lacrimal gland then pierces the septum and divides into two lateral palpebral branches in the lids.

The supraorbital artery joins the supraorbital nerve in the roof of the orbit and accompanies it through the supraorbital notch. It passes upwards deep to frontalis and its branches contribute to the supply of the forehead, scalp and upper lid.

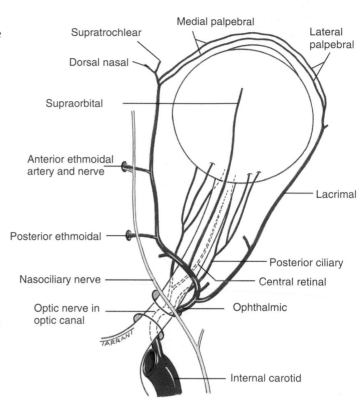

Diag. 1.10

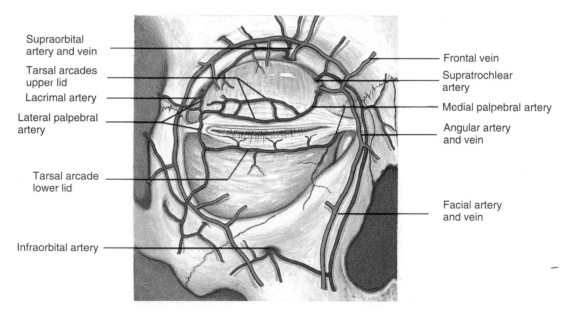

Diag. 1.11

The dorsal nasal artery pierces the septum above the medial canthal tendon to supply the skin of the root of the nose and the lacrimal sac. It often gives off the medial palpebral arteries although these may arise separately from the ophthalmic artery. The two medial palpebral arteries enter the lids above and below the medial canthal tendon.

In the lids the medial and lateral palpebral arteries anastomose to form tarsal arcades on the surface of the upper and lower tarsal plates 2–4 mm from the lid margins. In the upper lid a second arcade is formed at the upper border of the tarsal plate.

The supratrochlear artery pierces the septum with the supratrochlear nerve, winds upwards into the medial forehead and supplies it. It anastomoses with the supraorbital artery.

Blood from the external carotid system reaches the lids through anastomoses with the infraorbital and facial arteries, mainly via the angular artery, and the superficial temporal artery.

1.14b Venous drainage

The veins of the lids are found mainly in the region of the fornices (Diag. 1.11). They drain to the venous network of the middle third of the face.

The angular vein is formed by the anastomosis of the supraorbital and supratrochlear or frontal veins at the upper inner angle of the orbit. It drains posteriorly into the superior orbital vein and inferiorly into the facial vein. It lies about 8 mm medial to the inner canthus where it can often be seen through the skin.

Venous blood also drains to the inferior ophthalmic vein.

1.15 Lymphatic drainage of the lids
(Diag. 1.12)

The lateral two-thirds of the lids drain to the preauricular and parotid lymph nodes. The medial parts of the lids drain to the submandibular nodes.

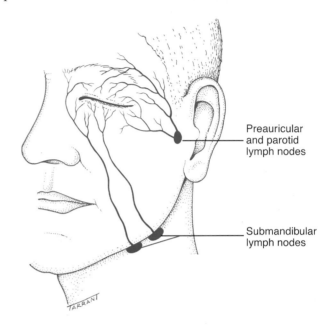

Preauricular and parotid lymph nodes

Submandibular lymph nodes

Diag. 1.12

1.16 Nerve supply to the lids and face

1.16a Motor supply

The muscles of facial expression, including orbicularis oculi, frontalis, procerus and corrugator supercilii develop from the second branchial arch and are supplied by the zygomatic branches of the facial nerve. The nerves travel deep to the muscles. Having reached the lids, they turn at right angles to the muscle bundles to approach the lid margins except medially where they run in the line of the muscles (Diag. 1.3).

The levator muscle is supplied by the third cranial nerve. The superior division of the nerve traverses and supplies the superior rectus muscle before supplying the levator.

Muller's muscle is supplied by sympathetic nerves probably travelling on the surface of arteries.

1.16b Sensory supply

The lids and the contents of the orbit are supplied by
the ophthalmic and maxillary divisions of the fifth
cranial nerve.

The ophthalmic division of the nerve divides in the
lateral wall of the cavernous sinus into the lacrimal,
frontal and nasociliary nerves. These pass through the
superior orbital fissure into the orbit.

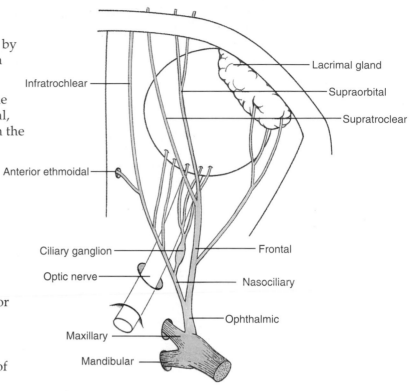

Diag. 1.13

The lacrimal nerve runs forward along the superior
border of the lateral rectus muscle to supply the
lacrimal gland. For its anterior two-thirds it is
accompanied by the lacrimal artery. It pierces the
septum and supplies sensation to the lateral part of
the upper lid and conjunctiva (Diag. 1.15). The
parasympathetic innervation of the lacrimal gland
travels with the zygomatic nerve from the spheno-
palatine ganglion and joins the lacrimal nerve just
posterior to the gland.

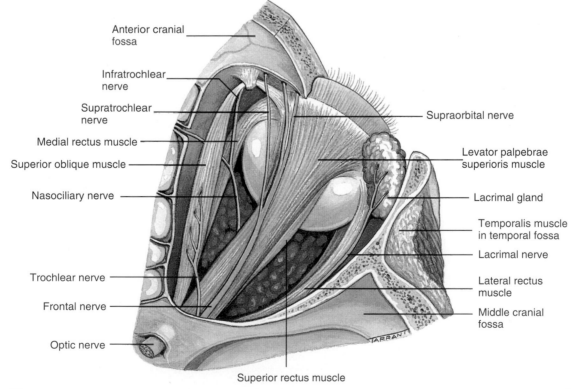

Diag. 1.14

The frontal nerve is the largest of the three branches. It passes forward between the periosteum of the orbital roof and the levator muscle. Anteriorly it divides into the supratrochlear and supraorbital nerves.

The supratrochlear nerve ascends over the medial orbital rim with the artery, deep to orbicularis, to supply the medial part of the lid and conjunctiva and the skin of the forehead. The supraorbital nerve continues to the supraorbital notch with the artery medial to it. It breaks into branches and supplies the upper lid and conjunctiva and the forehead and scalp as far as the vertex. It travels deep to orbicularis and frontalis and pierces them to reach the skin.

The nasociliary nerve crosses medially above the optic nerve with the ophthalmic artery. It gives origin to several branches then divides into the anterior ethmoidal nerve and the supratrochlear nerve. The anterior ethmoidal passes via the anterior cranial fossa to terminate as nasal nerves which supply the tip of the nose including the anterior part of the septum. The infratrochlear passes below the trochlea to supply the medial ends of the lids and conjunctiva, the lacrimal sac and root of the nose.

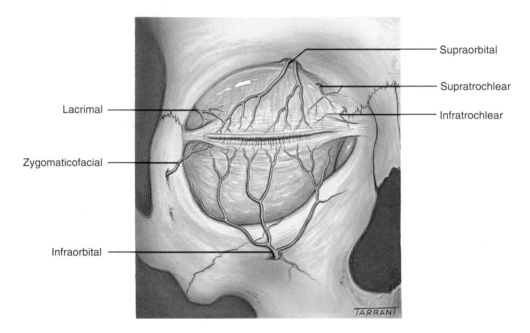

Supraorbital

Supratrochlear

Infratrochlear

Lacrimal

Zygomaticofacial

Infraorbital

Diag. 1.15

There are several communications between the terminal branches of the ophthalmic nerve around the eye. They also communicate with the infraorbital nerve, a branch of the maxillary division of the fifth cranial nerve.

The maxillary nerve passes forward from the trigeminal ganglion to the foramen rotundum through which it enters the pterygopalatine fossa. The infraorbital nerve branches forward and travels in a groove, then a canal, in the floor of the orbit to reach the infraorbital foramen. It branches to supply the skin and conjunctiva of the lower lid, the lower part of the side of the nose and the upper lip.

1.17 *The oriental eyelid*

The main difference from the occidental lid is the low skin crease due to the low insertion of the levator aponeurosis close to the lashes in the upper lid.

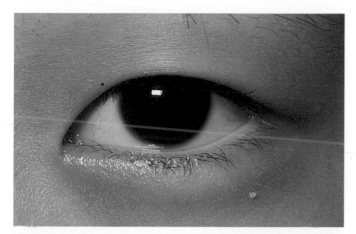

Fig. 1.5

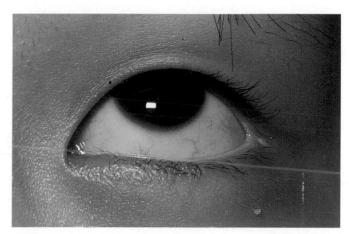

Fig. 1.6

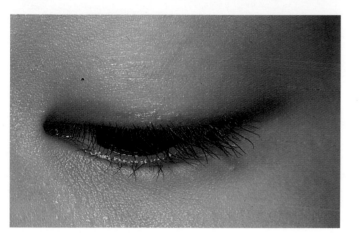

Fig. 1.7

The septum also inserts low on the aponeurosis. Both the fat in the retro-orbicular fascia and the preaponeurotic fat extend well down towards the lashes.

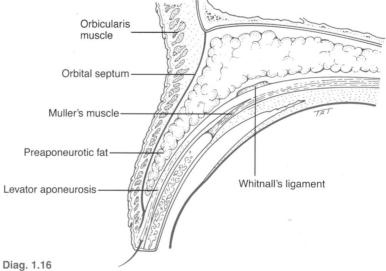

Diag. 1.16

1.18 Age changes in the lids

The lid and adnexal tissues lose tone and tissue bulk with age. The skin becomes loose and wrinkled as the collagen thins and the dermis becomes atrophic. Orbital fat atrophy causes a small and variable degree of enophthalmos. The orbital septum weakens and some fat prolapse may occur into the lids. The canthal tendons relax, the palpebral fissure shortens horizontally and the tension which holds the lids against the globe is gradually lost. An attenuated levator aponeurosis may stretch and lose its firm attachment to the tissues of the upper lid. The lower lid retractors may also become lax or disinsert from the lower tarsus.

The brows may droop as the epicranial aponeurosis stretches and the action of frontalis weakens. This adds to any redundant skin already present in the upper lid. Lacrimal secretion is reduced. Lost eyebrows and lashes are replaced less efficiently but they retain their pigmentation long after grey hair has appeared on the scalp.

These changes lead to many of the conditions which present to the ophthalmic plastic surgeon.

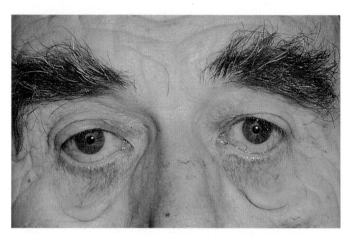

Fig. 1.9

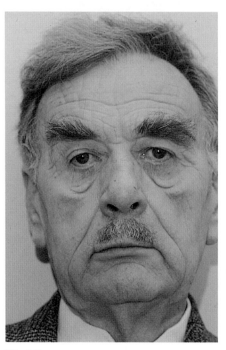

Fig. 1.8

FURTHER READING

Beard C, Quickert M H: Anatomy of the orbit (a dissection manual), 2nd ed. Aesculapius Publishing Company, Birmingham, Alabama; 1977

Doxanas M T, Anderson R L: Clinical orbital anatomy. Williams & Wilkins, Baltimore, Maryland; 1984

Doxanas M T, Anderson R L: Oriental eyelids. An anatomic study. Arch Ophthalmol 102: 1232; 1984

Koornneef L: Spatial aspects of orbital musculofibrous tissue in man. Swets and Seitlinger, Amsterdam; 1976

Lemke B N, Della Rocca R C: Surgery of the eyelids and orbit – an anatomical approach. Prentice Hall, New Jersey; 1990

Warwick R: Eugene Wolff's anatomy of the eye and orbit, 7th edn. H K Lewis, London; 1976

Zide B M, Jelks G W: Surgical anatomy of the orbit. Raven Press, New York; 1985

CHAPTER 2

Basic techniques in ophthalmic plastic surgery

Ophthalmic plastic surgery shares many basic techniques with general plastic surgery. During the past hundred years new techniques have been developed which take maximum advantage of the specialised anatomy of the eyelids and periorbital region.

The patient lies supine for ophthalmic plastic surgery and we find it helpful to stand to operate. By standing rather than sitting the surgeon can place himself in the best position for dissection and the placement of sutures. The drapes should leave both eyes exposed. Any standard skin preparation solution which is safe around the eyes may be used for ophthalmic plastic surgery. Aqueous povidone iodine 10% is safe but care is needed with aqueous chlorhexidine 1% which is toxic to the cornea.

At the end of the operation insert a traction suture if the lids are likely to open beneath the dressing (Fig 2.19), put antibiotic ointment into the eye and apply a dressing of a single layer of paraffin gauze and two eyepads onto the closed lids. Secure this with firm adhesive tape. The dressing in children, in particular, needs to be firmly secured if it is to stay in place.

Incisions

Scars are least obvious if incisions are made in or parallel to skin creases, the so-called relaxed skin tension lines, which form at right angles to the direction of action of the underlying muscle group and across which the tension is low (Diag. 2.1).

This general rule about the placement of incisions is modified in the lower lid when small lesions, not involving the lid margin, are excised. Unless there is an excess of loose skin the ellipse should be placed across the skin creases, at right angles to the lid margin, to avoid an ectropion.

The skin around the eyes is thin and mobile and it is helpful to stretch it along the intended incision line to ensure a clean cut at right angles to the skin. Incisions must be marked before distortions such as local anaesthetic infiltration or stretching are introduced.

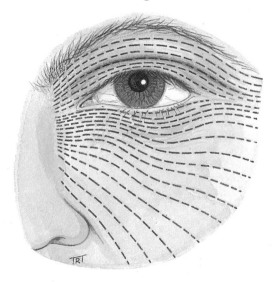

Diag. 2.1

Wound closure

2:1 Routine Wound Closure

Superficial wounds no deeper than the dermis and superficial subcutaneous fat may be closed with skin sutures alone. In deeper wounds subcutaneous absorbable sutures must usually be inserted to close the deep tissues to avoid a sunken scar.

Sutures in the range 4/0 to 7/0 are preferred. Non-absorbable interrupted or continuous sutures are used for skin closure but absorbable sutures are preferable in children.

Needle bites in each layer of the wound closure must be of equal depth on each side of the wound or a distorted closure will result. At the skin the needle should enter and leave at right angles. This will heap up the tissues slightly when the knots are tied and help to prevent a sunken scar.

Undermining the skin on either side of a wound will reduce tension across the closure. It is not necessary in most situations of simple wound closure. However, undermining is always necessary to create a skin flap. In the face the dissection should be in the fat just deep to the dermis to avoid damage to the facial nerve. Lift the wound edge to be undermined with skin hooks or a small retractor and dissect with a scalpel or scissors.

Closure of a wound may result in a dog-ear at one or both ends. Having closed the wound as far as possible insert a skin hook into the dog-ear and incise around its base to remove the unwanted skin.

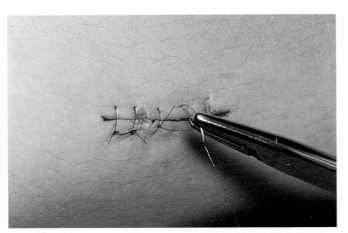

Fig. 2.1a

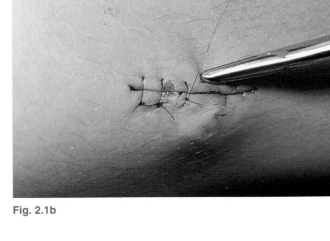

Fig. 2.1b

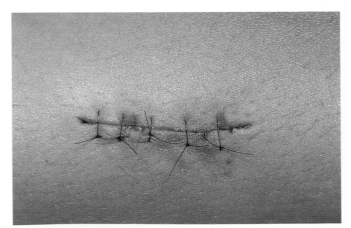

Fig. 2.1c

2:2 Mattress sutures

If there is a tendency for the skin edges to invert this can be overcome by the use of interrupted vertical mattress sutures.

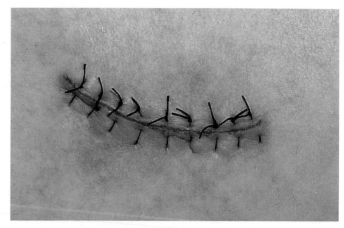

Fig. 2.2

2:3 Continuous sutures

If there is undue distortion at the skin edges from a simple 'over-and-over' continuous suture a continuous interlocking suture may be used instead.

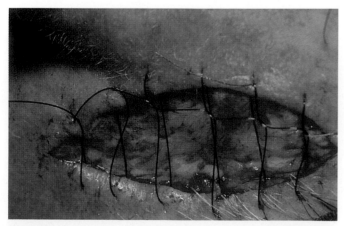

Fig. 2.3a

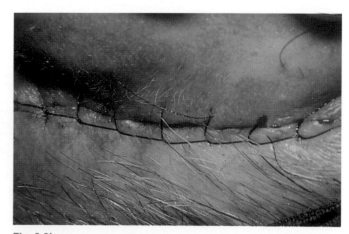

Fig. 2.3b

To avoid stitch marks a continuous intradermal suture allows adequate closure but a few interrupted sutures, or sterile adhesive dressing strips, may be needed to achieve perfect skin apposition.

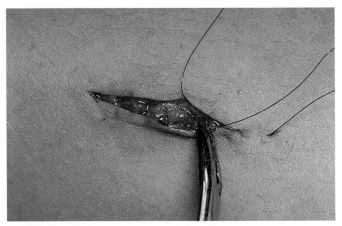

Fig. 2.4a

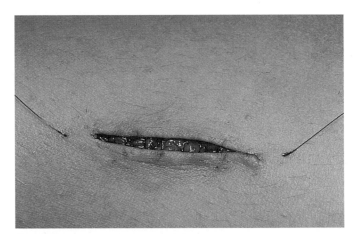

Fig. 2.4b

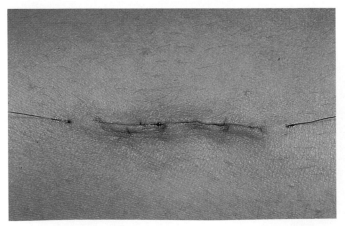

Fig. 2.4c

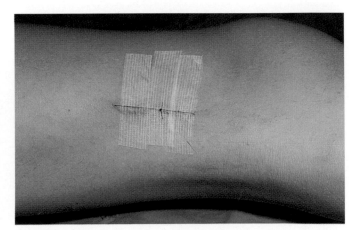

Fig. 2.4d

2:5 | **Three-point suture**

Where a V-shaped wound is to be closed or two wounds join at a T the 'three-point' suture is an effective method of closing the tip of the V or the junction at the T.

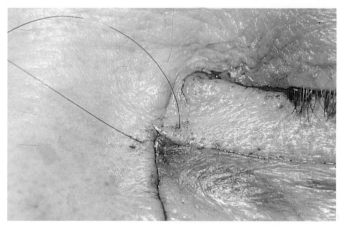

Fig. 2.5

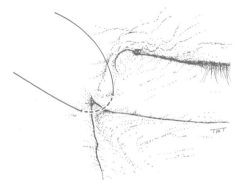

Key diag. 2.5

Complications and management

The healing process starting with an obvious hard, red scar and ending with a much less obvious soft, relatively avascular scar may take up to a year in adults and longer in children. It is usually quicker in the thin skin of the lids. If an unsightly scar persists massage often helps to hasten softening. It can be started after 10 days and should be gently but firmly applied for 5 minutes three times daily until the scar is seen to be soft. A lanolin ointment may be used at the time of massage. For management of a keloid scar see 2.18. A sunken or distorted scar can be avoided by accurate closure of the original wound. Once healed a poor scar must be excised and carefully resutured. Distortion due to contraction of a linear scar is corrected with a Z-plasty where possible.

2:6 Full thickness eyelid margin excision and repair

2.6a,b

2.6a,b Mark the first two cuts at right angles to the lid margin. Join them to form a pentagon of lid tissue to be excised. Use scissors to make the cuts. Bleeding will be mainly from the tarsal arcades which lie on the tarsal plates, close to the lid margins, in the upper and lower eyelids. In the upper lid a second arterial arcade lies just superior to the upper tarsal border. Pinch the full thickness of the lid gently with forceps either side of the wound to control the bleeding while the vessels are cauterised.

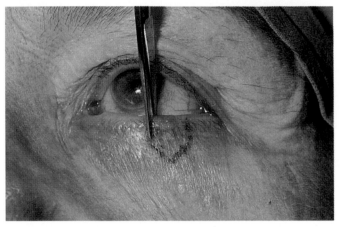

Fig. 2.6a

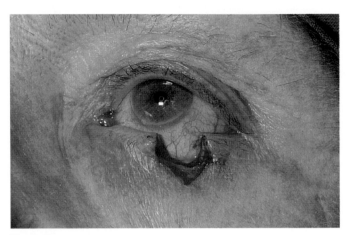

Fig. 2.6b

2.6c,d

Place a 6/0 or 7/0 absorbable suture through the cut edge of the tarsal plate close to the lid margin but avoid including the conjunctiva. Tie the knot on the anterior surface of the tarsus.

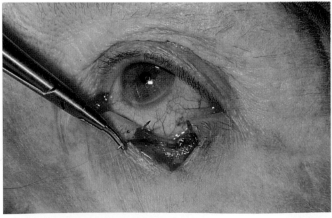

Fig. 2.6c

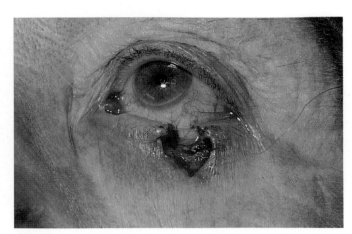

Fig. 2.6d

Full thickness eyelid margin excision and repair

2.6e

Place two more absorbable sutures through the remaining tarsal plate in the same way. Place a 6/0 silk suture through the grey line taking care that the needle enters and leaves at right angles to the lid margin. Leave the ends of this suture long.

Remove the skin sutures at 3 days and the grey line suture at a week. (See Figs 14.1d, 14.1 Post.)

Exactly the same steps are followed in the upper lid.

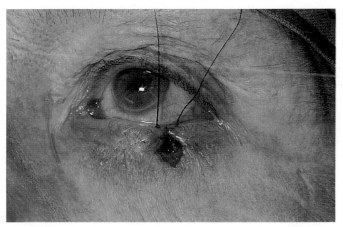

Fig. 2.6e

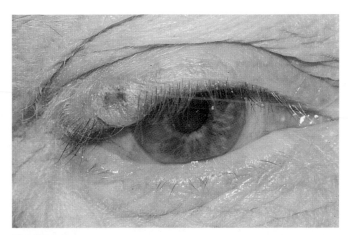

Fig. 2.6 pre

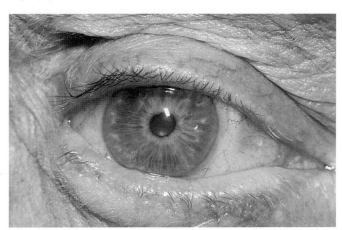

Fig. 2.6 post

2.6f

Close the orbicularis muscle with three 6/0 or 7/0 absorbable sutures. Close the skin with interrupted 6/0 silk sutures starting at the lash line. Use the uppermost suture to tie down the long end of the grey line suture.

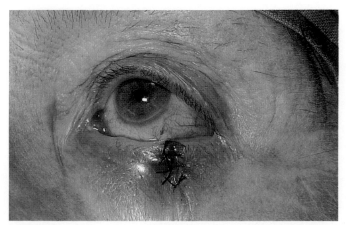

Fig. 2.6f

Complications and management

If the lid heals with a large notch excise the notch and resuture the lid.

Trichiasis may follow inaccurate closure with a notch. If the notch does not require excision treat the lashes with cryotherapy (see Ch. 8). Otherwise excise the area the resuture.

Skin grafts

2:7 | Postauricular skin

Skin from this site gives a good colour match with eyelid skin. In the preseptal part of the upper lid, however, skin from the opposite upper lid, or split skin, are preferable.

Taking full thickness grafts

2.7a

Cut a paper or foil template of the area to be grafted and mark out the graft behind the ear. It may be helpful to suture the pinna forward to the cheek. Inject saline subcutaneously to help in removal of the graft and to reduce bleeding. Adrenaline 1 : 200 000 will further reduce bleeding.

2.7b

Incise around the mark. Begin dissection of the graft superiorly. Hold the free edge of the graft with skin hooks, exerting gentle traction upwards with minimum bending of the graft. Dissect parallel to the skin with a rounded blade (e.g. No. 10 or No. 15 Bard Parker) and include as little of the subcutaneous tissue as possible. Secure haemostasis and close the skin with a continuous 4/0 interlocking suture (see 2.3). Remove this at 10 days.

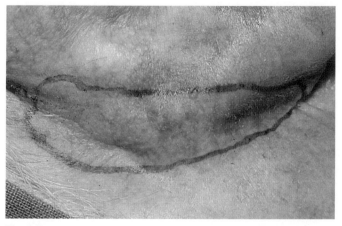

Fig. 2.7a

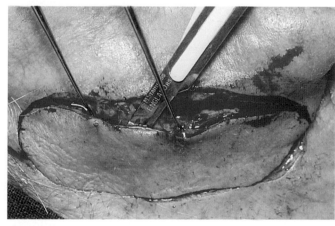

Fig. 2.7b

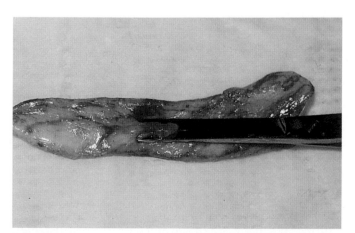

Fig. 2.7c

2.7c

A small amount of subcutaneous tissue is usually taken with the graft. It must be removed before the graft is used.

Complications and management

If there is difficulty closing the postauricular wound the skin over the mastoid may be undermined to achieve closure. The risk of poor vascularisation of the graft, with possible necrosis, is increased if the skin is thick or if the fat has been inadequately removed.

2:8   Upper lid skin

The ideal donor site for a graft to the upper lid is the
opposite upper lid. Upper lid skin can also be used in
the lower lid although it is thinner than lower lid skin.
Use a paper template of the recipient site to be grafted.
The graft is taken as for an upper lid blepharoplasty
and the same principles apply (see 10.1; Figs 7.7c, 7.7
Post, 15.1b,c).

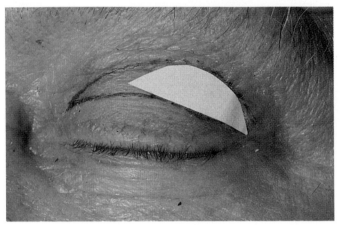

Fig. 2.8a

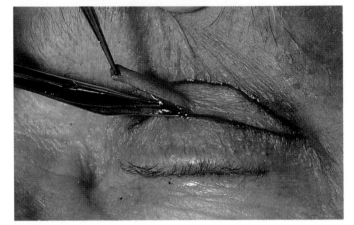

Fig. 2.8b

2:9   Preauricular skin

The skin immediately anterior to the tragus of the ear is
an alternative source of full thickness skin. It is thin
and readily accessible. A graft of up to 1×4 cm may be
obtained.

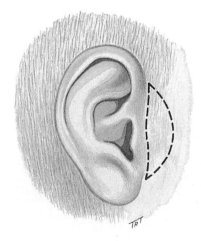

Diag. 2.2

Alternative sources of full thickness skin

Although inferior in colour match and texture, skin from the supraclavicular fossa or the antecubital fossa also may
be used in the periorbital region.

Taking a split skin graft

2:10a   Split skin grafts from arm or thigh

Split skin grafts may be taken from the inner aspect of the arm or thigh. Experience is needed to set the knife blade correctly if a Watson or Humby-style knife (see 5.10) is to be used. A blade clearance of 1/3–1/2 mm set by eye will give a suitable thickness. An alternative is to use a dermatome.

2.10a

Lubricate the knife blade and the edge of one of the two wooden boards with liquid paraffin. Apply firm traction to the skin with the lubricated board against the countertraction exerted by an assistant using the other board. Begin with the boards close together and apply the knife blade to the skin gently and at an angle. It is helpful for an assistant to press from the opposite side of the limb to create a larger flat area for the knife.

Using a to-and-fro movement in the line of the knife carefully begin to cut the graft, gently advancing the blade and at the same time moving your board away from the assistant's board, keeping firm traction on the skin to ensure a clean and accurate cut.

2.10b

Aim to cut a thin graft leaving multiple small points of haemorrhage on the cut surface. No fat should be visible. When a suitable graft has been cut the attached border can be most safely cut with fine scissors. Alternatively the Watson knife may be swept upwards to make the cut.

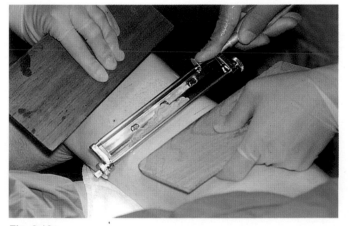

Fig. 2.10a

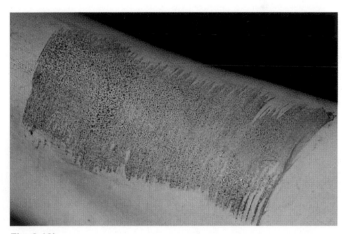

Fig. 2.10b

Technique continues overleaf ➔

Split skin grafts from arm or thigh

2.10c

Place the graft on paraffin gauze, cut surface uppermost, ready to be used. Dress the donor site with paraffin gauze and cover it with gauze and wool for 10–14 days. If leakage through the dressing occurs do not redress the donor site before 10 days but add extra dressing on top of the main dressing.

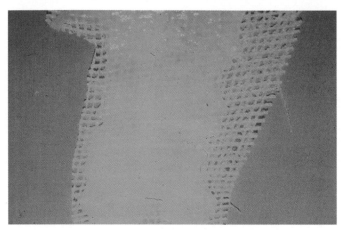

Fig. 2.10c

Complications and management

The graft may be cut too thickly, exposing an area of subcutaneous fat. Such an area will not heal like a split skin donor site by re-epithelialisation and it is best to cover it with split skin.

If there is difficulty removing the dressing from the donor site either leave the dressing to separate spontaneously over a week or so or soak it off.

Storage of skin grafts

Grafts of split or full thickness skin may be stored wrapped in sterile gauze moistened with Ringer's solution or saline at 4°C for a few days.

Skin graft fixation

It is usually necessary to apply fixed pressure to a graft for a week or so to immobilise it on its base and prevent tearing of the fine new vessels growing into it. In the lower lid, however, a simple pressure dressing left in place for 5 days is usually sufficient.

2:11 Graft stabilisation with a fixed bolster

2.11a

Place the graft, without tension, into the defect. Use 6/0 sutures to fix the graft, leaving alternate sutures long. Full thickness grafts are sutured edge to edge with surrounding skin. Split thickness grafts are draped over the edge of the surrounding skin and the sutures placed through the graft into the underlying skin edge. The peripheral fringe of split skin overlying the intact skin will not take. Small cuts may be made in the graft to allow blood to escape.

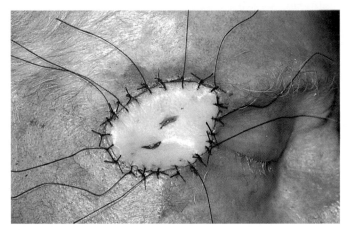

Fig. 2.11a

Graft stabilisation with a fixed bolster

2:12 Graft fixation with a pressure dressing

2.11b

Prepare a bolster of cotton wool. Soak it in flavine, if available, or saline and squeeze it out until just moist. Place a smooth surface of the bolster on the graft to apply even pressure. Fix the bolster in place with the long sutures tied together over it.

As an alternative, if no bolster is to be used with a lower lid graft, place simple sutures to fix the graft (see Fig. 16.4g). Apply a pressure dressing of paraffin gauze overlaid with moist cotton wool which can be moulded to the shape of the area. This is left undisturbed for 5 days.

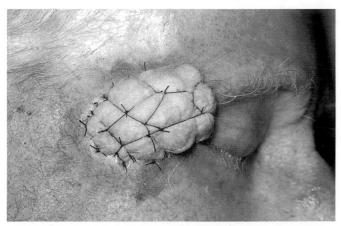

Fig. 2.11b

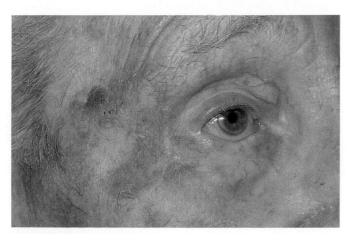

Fig. 2.11 post

Complications and management

A haematoma must be evacuated without delay if the area of the graft overlying it is to survive. Small incisions in the graft will help to prevent this occurring.

If infection occurs take immediate specimens for microscopy, culture and sensitivities. Treat *Streptococcus pyogenes* or *Pseudomonas pyocyanea*. Treat other pathogens if the infection is marked. Assess the appearance of the graft – often more survives than seems likely at first. If a large area of the graft fails regraft with split skin on clean granulation tissue, free of slough, after about 3 weeks.

Graft contraction is more of a problem with split skin than full thickness skin. Allowance for contraction must be made when a graft is planned. Repeat grafting may be necessary to overcome the effects of contraction. This can be done as needed at any time after 3 weeks.

If the graft becomes ischaemic wait for 3–6 weeks. Often more of the graft survives than seems likely at first. If a large area of the graft fails allow the necrotic area to separate and regraft this area with split skin at about 3 weeks when granulations have formed. Prevent infection with antibiotic powder. Necrosis is usually due to haematoma formation under the graft or to infection. However, if the graft is thick or the fat has been inadequately removed the risk of ischaemia increases. To cover a site of previous irradiation a flap is preferable to a graft.

Grafts for reconstruction of the posterior eyelid lamella

2:13   Taking an oral mucous membrane graft

Mucous membrane grafts of up to about 3×1.5cm may be taken safely from the lower lip. Larger grafts may be taken from the cheek having identified the opening of the parotid duct at the level of the crown of the second upper molar tooth. (See Figs 6.6b, 15.3c.)

2.13a

2.13a While an assistant holds the lip or cheek firmly in a gauze estimate the area of mucosa needed, allowing some excess for later contraction. Mark the graft, avoiding the vermilion border of the lip, and inject saline or 1:200 000 adrenaline into the submucosal tissues to give some rigidity and to reduce bleeding.

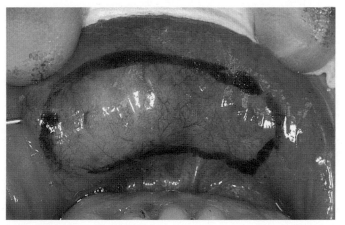

Fig. 2.13a

2.13b

Cut around the mark to the level of the submucosa. Dissect the graft from the submucosal tissues with scissors or a blade holding the upper edge with skin hooks. There is usually moderate bleeding. Take care not to remove mucosa too far down into the gingival fossa, particularly if the patient wears dentures.

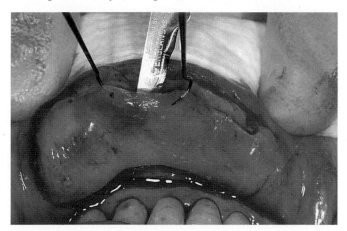

Fig. 2.13b

2.13c

Secure haemostasis. The bed of the graft will heal well without sutures but a continuous 4/0 absorbable suture may be used to close the defect. Prescribe frequent mouthwashes postoperatively.

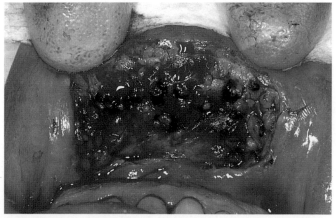

Fig. 2.13c

Technique continues overleaf ➜

Taking an oral mucous membrane graft

2:14 Split thickness mucous membrane grafts

2.13d

Remove any submucosal tissue from the graft before use.

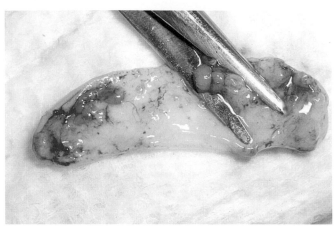

Fig. 2.13d

Split thickness oral mucosa is preferable for replacing bulbar conjunctiva because it is thinner and looks less erythematous. The technique is as for a full thickness graft but a split thickness graft is taken with a Castroviejo mucotome or a Silver's skin graft knife.

2:15 Preparation of donor sclera

Sclera is a readily available and convenient material for use as a spacer. It contracts more than cartilage and is less rigid.

Clean the surface of a donor eye, remove the cornea, evaginate the eye and clean away all tissue down to the sclera. Store the sclera at 4°C in 10% buffered formaldehyde solution or 70% alcohol.

Before use wash it in about six changes of saline over 24 hours and soak it in antibiotic solution for 2 hours. Mark and cut the sclera to the appropriate size. (See also Figs 11.4b, 11.7d, 13.1a, 13.2a.)

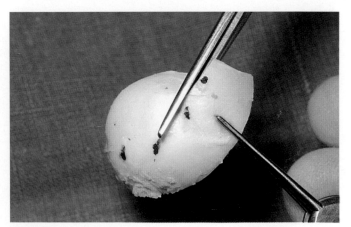

Fig. 2.15

Complications and management

A shallowed gingival fossa is not serious unless the patient wears dentures which can no longer be worn with comfort. New dentures may be needed.

Damage to the vermilion border of the lip may result from an attempt to take too large a graft. Healing will usually occur without complication.

Damage to the parotid duct results from the graft excision being taken too far posteriorly. Providing there is free drainage of parotid secretions into the mouth the duct will continue to function.

2:16 Taking auricular cartilage

Cartilage from the ear is more rigid than donor sclera but thinner than nasal septal cartilage.

2.16a

Hold the ear forward and mark the furrow between the two main areas of cartilage. Inject adrenaline 1:200 000 into the firm subcutaneous tissues to raise the skin away from the cartilage.

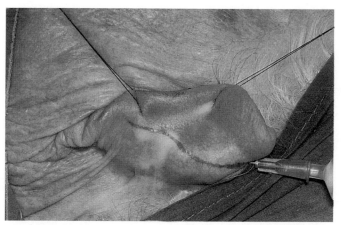

Fig. 2.16a

2.16b

Incise the skin at the mark and reflect it towards either the mastoid or the periphery of the ear, dissecting between the perichondrium and the cartilage. Leave the main ridge of cartilage of the antihelix intact at the site of the skin incision.

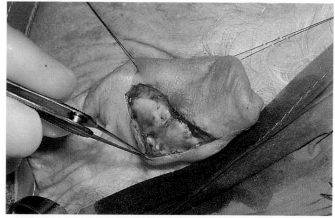

Fig. 2.16b

2.16c

Mark the area of cartilage to be excised. Make a partial thickness cut with a knife and complete it with a Rollett's rougine to enter the space between the anterior surface of the cartilage and its perichondrium. Dissect out the required cartilage and excise it.

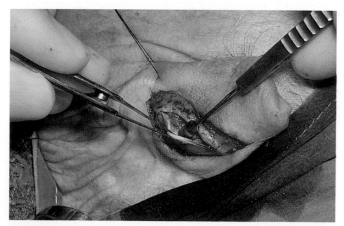

Fig. 2.16c

Technique continues overleaf →

Taking auricular cartilage

2.16d

Close the skin with a 4/0 mattress suture. Insert a small drain if there is residual bleeding.

Dress with a well-padded dressing. Remove the drain at 2 days and the suture at 10 days.

Complications and management

Postoperative swelling is usually marked and it settles spontaneously.

If a large haematoma forms it should be evacuated. Small haematomas are not uncommon and usually settle without problems.

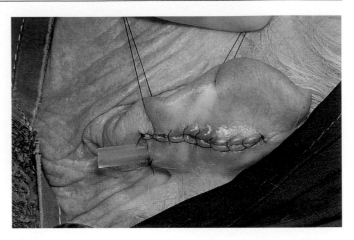

Fig. 2.16d

2:17 Taking a tarsal graft

Full thickness tarsal plate from the upper lid is an excellent posterior lamellar graft or spacer, with a mucosal lining, when only a small area is required. It may be taken from the ipsilateral or the contralateral side. (See Figs 15.5b, 15.6c.)

2.17a

Evert the upper lid over a Desmarres retractor and insert a stay suture close to the lid margin. Measure 4 mm from the lid margin at several points and mark off along this line the length of graft required.

2.17b

Incise the full thickness of the tarsal plate along the mark. Make vertical cuts from the ends of the first incision to the superior border of the tarsal plate and extend them for 2 mm into the conjunctiva. Undermine and excise the graft with about 2 mm of conjunctiva attached. Leave the donor site to granulate.

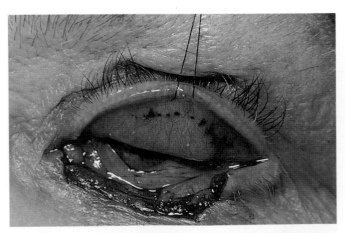

Fig. 2.17a

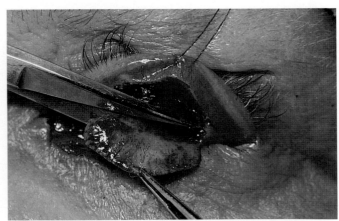

Fig. 2.17b

Other techniques

2:18   Taking autogenous fascia lata

2.18a

Make a straight incision 3–4 cm long in a line from the anterior superior iliac spine to the head of the fibula. The lower end of the incision should be about 5 cm above the knee joint.

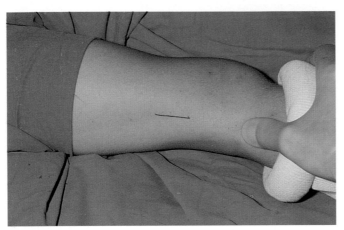

Fig. 2.18a

2.18b

Deepen the incision through the subcutaneous fat to expose the white, vertically striated ileotibial tract – the thickened lateral part of the fascia lata. Make two short parallel incisions 1 cm apart in the line of the fascial bands.

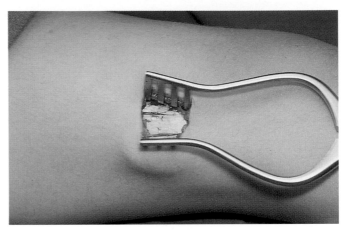

Fig. 2.18b

2.18e

Insert the end of the strip of fascia into the fasciotome.

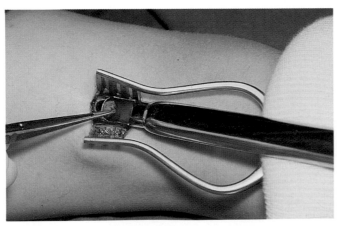

Fig. 2.18e

2.18f

Place two artery clips on its distal end. Keeping firm tension downwards on the fascia advance the fasciotome up the leg. Initial resistance may be encountered. Firm but careful manipulation of the

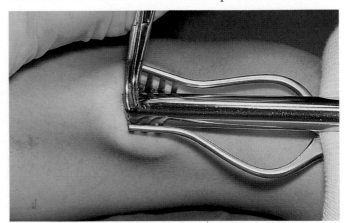

Fig. 2.18f

Taking autogenous fascia lata

2.18c

Using large straight Mayo scissors dissect the fascia free from the superficial and deep tissues above the wound by spreading the blades. Now with the scissors blades just open extend the first two parallel incisions upwards for a few centimetres in the line of the fascial bands.

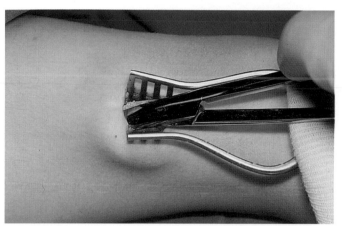

Fig. 2.18c

2.18d

Cut the fascia transversely to join the lower ends of the incisions and dissect the flap of fascia from the underlying muscle.

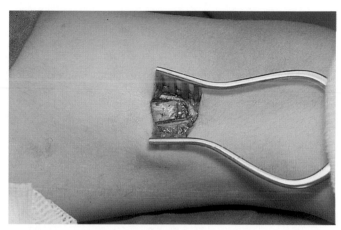

Fig. 2.18d

fasciotome while keeping downward tension on the fascia usually allows it to proceed into less difficult tissues. After this the progress is usually easier and the fasciotome should be advanced as far as possible. The strip of fascia created by this manoeuvre must now be separated at its proximal end. This is achieved in different ways depending on the fasciotome being used. With the Moseley fasciotome the inner part is pulled firmly back in relation to the outer part which is held steady. This cuts the fascia which should be kept under tension while it is being cut.

2.18g

Remove the fasciotome and the strip of fascia lata from the wound. Close the wound in two layers with a 4/0 absorbable subcutaneous suture and a 4/0 subcuticular suture or interrupted sutures.

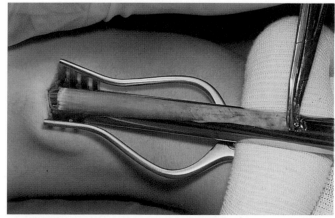

Fig. 2.18g

Technique continues overleaf →

Taking autogenous fascia lata

An eyelid commonly requires 1 or 2 days of postoperative traction either to maintain its position during the early healing phase or to protect the cornea beneath the dressing (the 'Frost' suture).

2.18h

Preparation of fascia lata – for ptosis surgery cut the fascia lata in the line of its fibres to create four strips about 2 mm in width. Avoid cutting across the fibres as this will weaken the strip. Place the cut strips and any spare fascia lata in saline.

2.19a,b

Insert a 4/0 or 6/0 silk suture through the grey line at the lid margin and out onto the skin 2–3 mm from the lashes. Pass it through a short length of tarsorrhaphy tubing then back through the skin and grey line. A small haemorrhage from the vascular arcade is common and can be ignored. Tape the suture to the brow (for the lower lid) or the cheek (for the upper lid) with sufficient traction to close the lid.

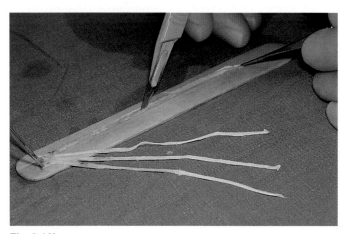

Fig. 2.18h

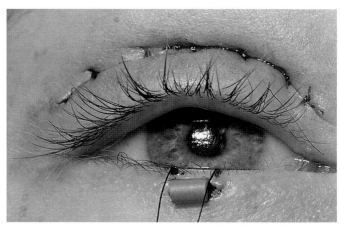

Fig. 2.19a

Complications and management

The leg scar is often obvious and may become hypertrophic or keloid. Injection of triamcinolone into the keloid, repeated several times if necessary, will flatten the scar. Care is needed in the use of this powerful steroid. An alternative is to apply constant pressure to the scar beneath a dressing. It may take several months before the scar is flattened.

Uncommonly, a small hernia of muscle may appear through the defect in the fascia lata. This should be left unless there is a significant problem.

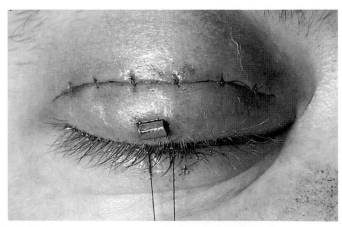

Fig. 2.19b

2:20   The Z-plasty

This technique is used either to overcome the effect of a contracted linear scar (see 7.6) or to break up the line of an obvious and unsightly scar (see 14.3). Thus the two results of any Z-plasty are first to lengthen the stem of the Z and secondly to rotate the stem of the Z. The angle of rotation will be 90 degrees if the limbs of the Z are at 60 degress to the stem.

Since no extra tissue is being introduced by a Z-plasty the lengthening effect in one direction is bought at the expense of tissue shortening at right angles.

If the scar is long it is preferable to create two or more smaller Z-plasties along it rather than one large one. This results in a less obvious scar and the tension at right angles to the Z is less.

Mark the linear scar A–B (see Diag. 2.3) and measure its length. This will be the stem of the Z. Draw a line from each end equal in length to the stem and at 60 degrees to it. Take time to plan the direction of the two end lines. In some situations they will obviously 'fit' better on the opposite side of the stem.

Create the stem of the Z-plasty by excising the scar. Incise the remainder of the Z and undermine the flaps c and d (see Diag. 2.3) widely enough to allow them to be transposed without obvious tension. Excise any remaining deep scar tissue revealed by reflecting the flaps.

Subcutaneous sutures of 6/0 catgut may be needed if the flaps are relatively thick. Usually, however, skin sutures alone are adequate.

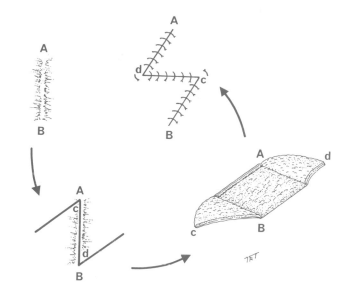

Diag. 2.3

Complications and management

If necrosis occurs at the tips of the flaps, wait – the colour often improves with survival of all of the flap skin. If a large area does necrose a full thickness skin graft onto clean granulations at about 3 weeks will usually take well.

Continuing distortion in the tissues is usually due to poor design of the Z-plasty or to the inappropriate use of a Z-plasty when a skin graft should have been used. In either case allow the area to heal and reassess it at 6 months.

FURTHER READING

Callahan M A, Callahan A (eds): Ophthalmic plastic and orbital surgery. Aesculapius Publishing Company, Birmingham, Alabama; 1979.

McGregor I A: Fundamental techniques in plastic surgery, 8th edn. Churchill Livingstone, Edinburgh; 1989.

Obvious pathology

Check the visual acuity.

Look for scars, inflammation, tumours and any other obvious abnormality. Record accurately the size, site and attachment to deeper structures.

Eyelid position

With the patient's eyes open look for ptosis or lid retraction (3.1), entropion, ectropion, telecanthus (3.2) and rounding or medial displacement of the lateral canthus.

| 3:1 | **Margin-reflex distance** |

3.1a

While the patient looks at an examination torch held about half a metre away measure the distance of each upper and lower lid from the corneal light reflex.

3.1b

This allows an accurate assessment of the relative positions of each of the four eyelids. It provides more information than a simple measurement of the vertical palpebral apertures because an inaccurate record of the position of the upper lids occurs if the lower lids are not level with each other. The margin-reflex distance (MRD) reveals this.

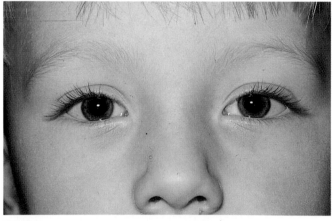

Fig. 3.1a

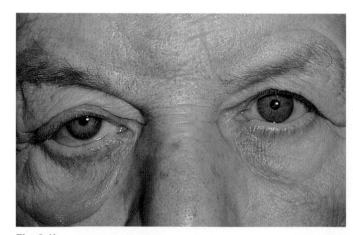

Fig. 3.1b

| 3:2 | **Telecanthus** |

The normal intercanthal distance is approximately half the interpupillary distance.

Eyelid movement

Check that the lids open and close normally and move normally in upgaze and downgaze. Assess levator function (3.3), the power of the orbicularis oculi and frontalis muscles and Bell's phenomenon (3.5). Look for jaw-winking (3.6).

3:3 Levator function

3.3a,b

Fix the brow with a thumb and measure the excursion of the upper lid between upgaze and downgaze.

Repeat two or three times on each side to check. Normal levator function is 12–15 mm.

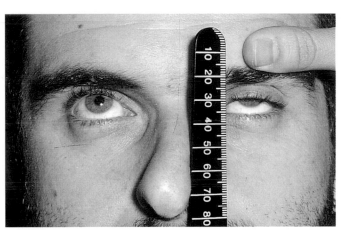

Fig. 3.3a

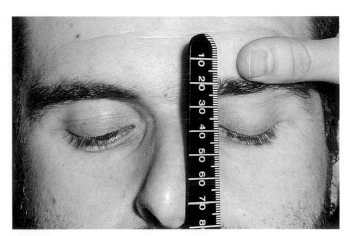

Fig. 3.3b

3.3c,d

Children may need something to watch and it may be helpful to hold the rule and the brow together leaving the other hand free.

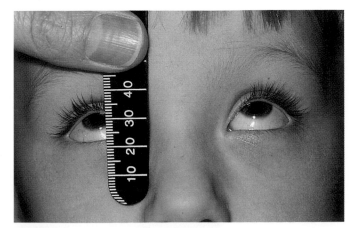

Fig. 3.3c

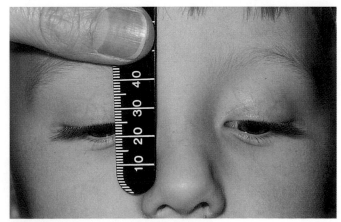

Fig. 3.3d

3:7   Fatigue in myasthenia gravis

Ask the patient to look up, without blinking, for 30 seconds. The upper lids will droop to a variable degree if fatigue is present.

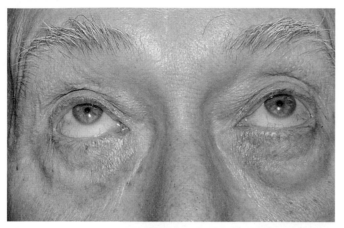

Fig. 3.7a

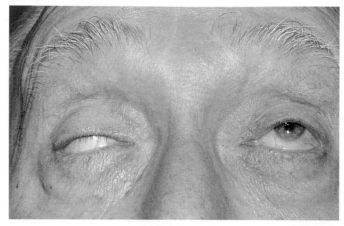

Fig. 3.7b

Eye position

Look for proptosis (3.8) or any vertical or horizontal displacement of either eye (3.9).

3:8   Exophthalmometry

3.8a,b

To make an approximate assessment of proptosis stand behind the patient and observe the relative position of the eyes from above.

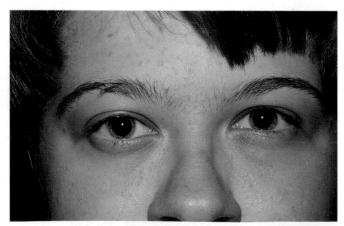

Fig. 3.8a

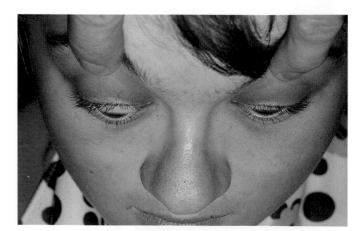

Fig. 3.8b

Exophthalmometry

3.8c

3.8c The Hertel exophthalmometer allows a much more accurate measurement to be made. Place the instrument on the lateral orbital rims and ask the patient to look directly ahead. Line up the mires and note the point on the scale cut by the reflection of the patient's corneas. Take several readings. Even so the error of the instrument is + or − 2 mm.

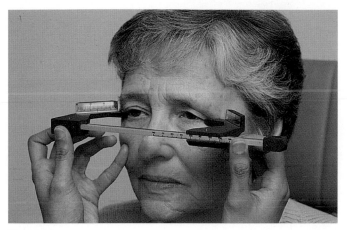

Fig. 3.8c

3:9   **Eye displacement**

Place a ruler horizontally level with the inferior limbus of one eye and check that the opposite eye is level. Measure the distance from the mid-point of the bridge of the nose to the corneal light reflex of each eye.

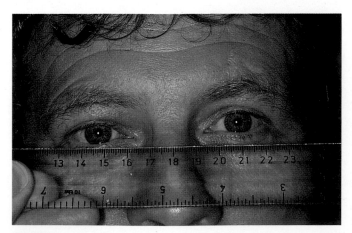

Fig. 3.9

Eye movement

Check the eye movements individually and together.

Other

It is convenient to start the other examinations at the brows and move down.

3:10   **Brow position**

Check that there is no brow ptosis. This is particularly important in the preoperative assessment before a blepharoplasty (see Ch. 10.)

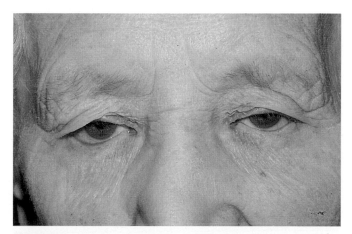

Fig. 3.10a

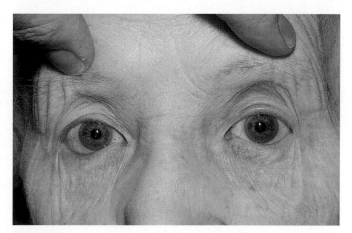

Fig. 3.10b

3:11 Upper lid skin crease

Measure the level of the upper lid skin crease from the centre of the lash line in each upper lid.

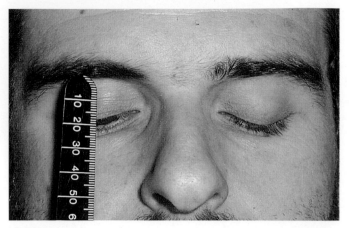

Fig. 3.11

3:12 Horizontal lower lid laxity

3.12a

Gently grasp the skin in the centre of the lower lid and pull the lid away from the eye. Abnormal laxity exists if the distance from the cornea to the posterior lid margin exceeds about 10 mm.

3.12b

Alternatively, place a finger on the centre of the inferior orbital rim and pull the lid away from the globe. Ask the patient not to blink and observe the speed of return of the lid back to the globe. A quick 'snap back' indicates minimal or no laxity. A slow return suggests mild laxity. Incomplete return unless the patient blinks suggests moderate laxity and in severe laxity there is incomplete return even after a blink.

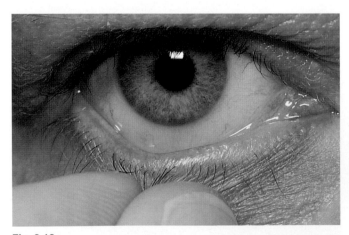

Fig. 3.12a

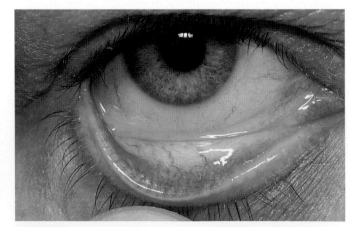

Fig. 3.12b

Horizontal lid laxity is due mainly, perhaps entirely, to laxity in one or both canthal tendons. This may occur alone or in combination with laxity in the orbicularis muscle.

3:13   **Medial and lateral canthal tendons**

3.13a

To assess the medial canthal tendon pull the lid laterally and observe the migration of the punctum. It should be just lateral to the caruncle at rest and it should move laterally no more than 1–2 mm. If it does, abnormal laxity is present.

3.13b

The lateral canthus should be 1–2 mm medial to the lateral orbital rim at rest. It should move medially no more than 1–2 mm with medial traction. Rounding of the normally sharp lateral canthus occurs if there is marked laxity of the tendon. It can be tested in a similar way to the medial canthal tendon.

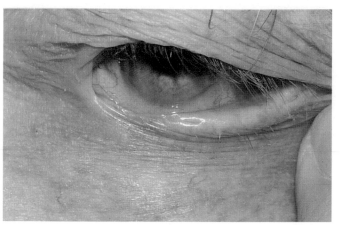

Fig. 3.13a

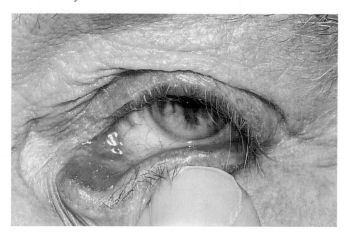

Fig. 3.13b

3:14   Eye and orbit

Check the visual acuity if not already done. Examine the external eye and the conjunctiva, particularly the tarsal conjunctiva of the upper and lower lids. Look for scarring and evidence of reduced tear production (3.14a,b). Palpate the anterior orbit for masses and the principal sites of lymph drainage for enlarged nodes. Where relevant measure the intraocular pressures and examine the fundi.

3.14a

Inadequate tear production is identified by fine punctate staining of the conjunctiva with Rose Bengal eye drops.

3.14b

The Schirmer filter paper test quantifies tear production. Instill local anaesthetic drops and measure the excursion of tears along the papers after 5 minutes – 10 mm or more may be considered adequate.

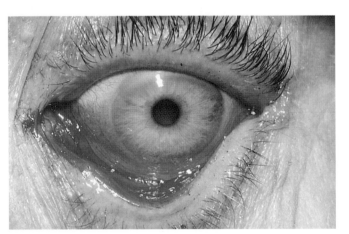

Fig. 3.14a

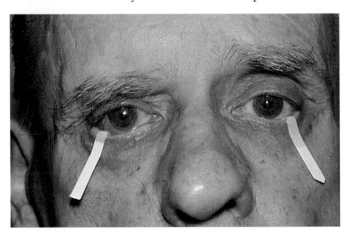

Fig. 3.14b

Photography

It is useful to keep a photographic record of the preoperative and postoperative appearances in most ophthalmic plastic cases. A macro lens capable of 1:1 magnification and with a focal length of about 100 mm is appropriate. Flash illumination is versatile with the exposure determined by either a manual setting or with through-the-lens (TTL) flash metering. 100ASA film is a convenient speed.

The most useful fields of view will be one eye (about 1:1), both eyes (about 1:3–1:4) and the whole face (about 1:10.)

Always obtain the patient's permission before taking photographs.

CHAPTER 4

Anaesthesia

Local anaesthesia is very satisfactory for most ophthalmic plastic procedures. Children and some adults require general anaesthesia. Extensive procedures are more conveniently done under general anaesthesia because of the volume of local anaesthetic which would be required.

Premedication

A mild sedative may be beneficial for anxious patients having surgery under local anaesthesia. Temazepam 10 mg orally 2 hours before operation is usually sufficient. The effect is less prolonged than diazepam but day patients are advised not to travel home alone if they have had premedication.

Local anaesthesia

Anaesthetic eye drops such as amethocaine 1% or oxybuprocaine 0.4% (Benoxinate) are given before skin preparation.

Lignocaine (xylocaine, lidocaine) 2% with 1:200 000 adrenaline gives excellent anaesthesia for local infiltration or regional block. After injection the anaesthetic is effective within 5 minutes and lasts an hour or so. A mixture of equal volumes of lignocaine and bupivicaine 0.5% (Marcaine) prolongs the anaesthesia. The addition of hyaluronidase promotes diffusion of the anaesthetic but increases its absorption and is generally not necessary.

Local infiltration

4:1   Subcutaneous

Having marked the incision inject local anaesthetic slowly into the subcutaneous layer (and the submuscular layer for deeper dissection) deep to the mark. Large volumes are not required and they distort the tissues.

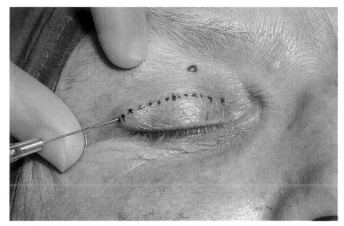

Fig. 4.1

4:2   Subconjunctival

4.2

If a posterior approach is used inject deep to the conjunctiva along the proximal border of the tarsal plate.

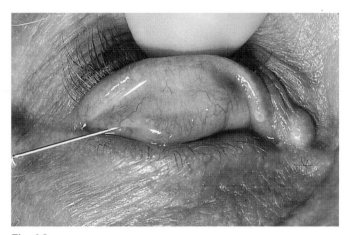

Fig. 4.2

As the operation proceeds extra anaesthetic may be given if sensation begins to return or if the surgery extends into an area not reached by the initial injection.

4:4　Infratrochlear nerve block

Anaesthesia of the medial end of the upper lid, side of the nose, medial conjunctiva, caruncle and lacrimal sac.

Pass the needle along the medial orbital wall from a point 1 cm superior to the medial canthus. Advance it 1.5cm and inject 2–3ml of anaesthetic.

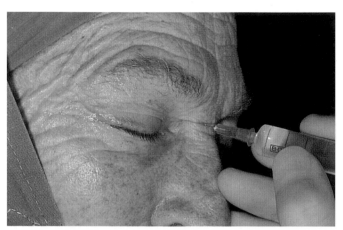

Fig. 4.4

4:5　Infraorbital nerve block

Anaesthesia of the skin and conjunctiva of the lower lid, the lower part of the side of the nose and part of the upper lip.

The infraorbital nerve emerges onto the cheek from the foramen 0.5–1 cm below the junction of the medial one-third and the lateral two-thirds of the inferior orbital rim. Inject 2–3ml of anaesthetic subcutaneously at this site to infiltrate around the nerve. This is a safer procedure than an attempt to enter the infraorbital foramen.

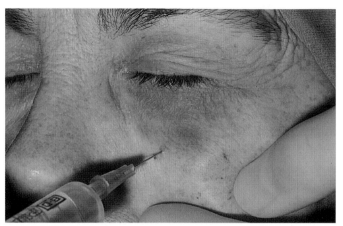

Fig. 4.5

4:6　Retrobulbar nerve block

Motor and sensory block of the contents of the orbit.

This block may be used for procedures such as enucleation if local anaesthesia is preferred.

From the junction of the middle and lateral thirds of the inferior orbital rim advance the needle over the rim for about 3cm, aiming at the apex of the orbit. Inject 2.0–3.0ml of anaesthetic.

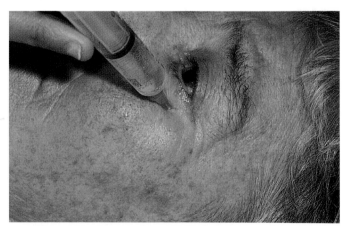

Fig. 4.6

4:7 Facial nerve block

This block is occasionally useful to prevent excessive movement of the facial muscles during lid procedures.

4.7a

Motor block of the trunk of the facial nerve.
From a point immediately anterior to the notch inferior to the tragus of the ear advance the needle until the ramus of the mandible is felt. Slightly withdraw the needle, tilt it posteriorly and advance just posterior to the ramus. Inject 2 ml of anaesthetic.

4.7b

Motor block of the branches to orbicularis oculi. Infiltrate anaesthetic subcutaneously and submuscularly just lateral to the lateral orbital rim.

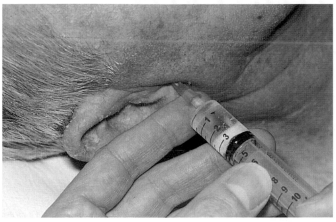

Fig. 4.7a

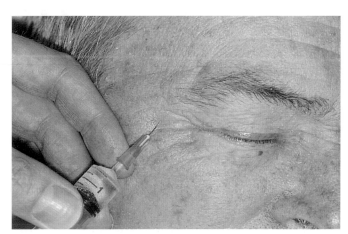

Fig. 4.7b

5:1   The basic instruments

The basic instruments

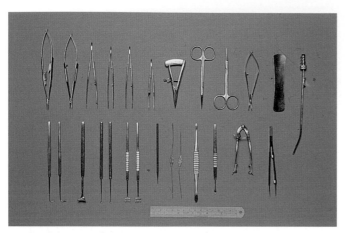

Fig. 5.1

Top row, left to right:
    Castroviejo needle holders
    Barraquer needle holders
    Jayle's forceps
    Lister's forceps
    Moorfield's forceps
    St Martin's forceps
    Measuring caliper
    Blunt-ended dissecting scissors
    Sharp-ended dissecting scissors
    Curved spring scissors
    Corneal guard spatula
    Fine sucker

Bottom row, left to right:
    Muscle hooks
    Desmarres retractor
    Skin hooks
    Catspaw retractors
    Nettleship punctal dilator
    Lacrimal probes
    Blunt dissector
    Rollet's rougine
    Eyelid speculum
    Bipolar diathermy forceps
    Rule

5:2   Detail of forceps

Top to bottom:
    St Martin's
    Jayle's
    Lister's
    Moorfield's

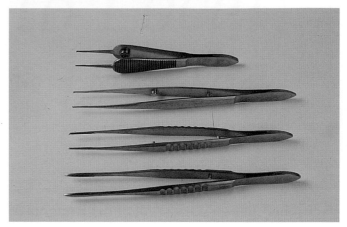

Fig. 5.2

5:3   Pen, scalpel, blades

Skin marking pen

Disposable scalpel with blades nos 15, 10 and 11

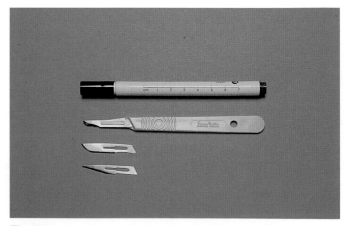

Fig. 5.3

5:4   Commonly used sutures

Top row: non-absorbable sutures
Bottom row: absorbable sutures

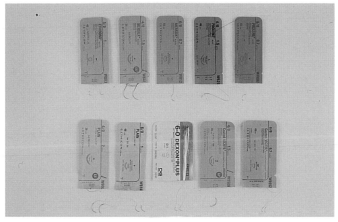

Fig. 5.4

5:6   Fascia lata set

Wright's fascia lata needle
Mayo scissors
Small self-retaining retractor
Small straight needle holder
Gillies' needle holder
Moseley fasciotome (parts separated)

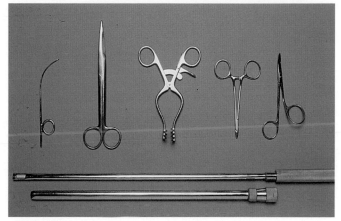
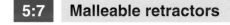

Fig. 5.6

5:5   Nasal speculum and bone punches

Nasal speculum
Sphenoidal bone punches
Compound action bone nibbler

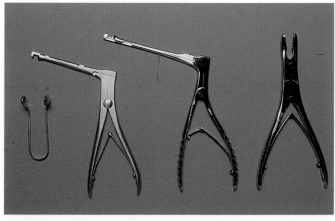

Fig. 5.5

5:7   Malleable retractors

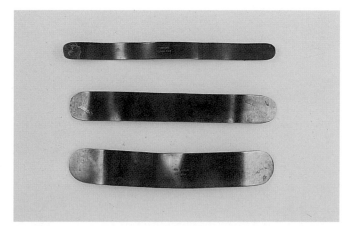

Fig. 5.7

5:8   Transnasal wire set

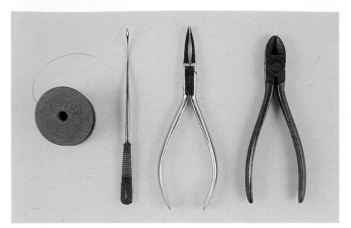

Stainless steel wire
Awl
Wire forceps
Wire cutters

Fig. 5.8

5:9   Air-powered oscillating saw with blades

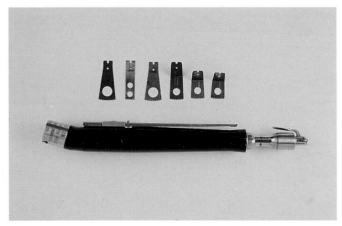

Fig. 5.9

5:10   Watson split skin knife with blade and boards

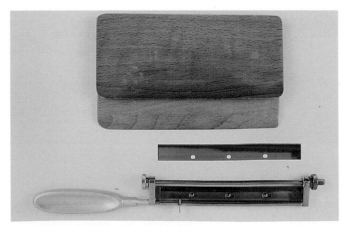

Fig. 5.10

See also the Crookshank clamp (6.11a).

CHAPTER 6

Entropion

Entropion of the upper or lower eyelids causes pain and leads eventually to corneal scarring. The changes occur more rapidly if there is also a poor tear film.

Classification: Involutional
Cicatricial
Congenital

Look for cicatricial changes in the conjunctiva. If present try to establish the cause before considering surgery (Section B).

If cicatricial changes are absent look for the transverse ridge of muscle caused by preseptal orbicularis overriding pretarsal orbicularis in the lower lid in involutional entropion (Section A).

Congenital entropion (Section C) is rare. It is diagnosed by complete inturning of the lid margin and tarsal plate.

Epiblepharon is common. The tarsal plate is in a normal position but a fold of skin and muscle, especially medially, cause the lashes to turn in. Epiblepharon usually requires no treatment.

Involutional entropion

Choice of operation

Assess the horizontal laxity in the lower lid (see 3.12).

If it is minimal a simple suture repair (6.1) is effective but may be temporary, lasting about 18 months. A lasting correction is more certain with the Wies procedure (6.2) which corrects more of the aetiological factors in involutional entropion.

If significant horizontal laxity is present assess the canthal tendons (see 3.13).

If either is very lax it must be stabilised first (see 7.4, 7.5, 7.9).

If only mild or moderate laxity of the canthal tendons is present or if there is residual laxity after one or both have been stabilised, choose the Quickert procedure (6.3).

The Jones procedure (6.4) tightens the lower lid retractors. It is used for recurrent involutional entropion if there is no other obvious cause.

6:1 Sutures

6.1a

Inject local anaesthetic subcutaneously and subconjunctivally. Place three double-armed 4/0 catgut sutures through the full thickness of the lateral two-thirds of the lid. Each suture is passed obliquely from 1 to 2mm inferior to the lower tarsal border to emerge 4mm inferior to the lashes. If the entropion is very mild the sutures may be passed horizontally through the lid immediately inferior to the tarsus to emerge in the skin at the same level as the entry into the conjunctiva.

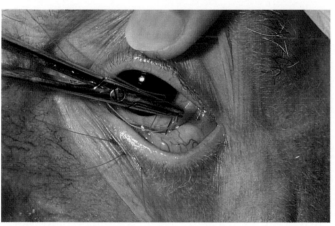

Fig. 6.1a

6.1b

Tie the sutures just tightly enough to produce a slight ectropion of the lid. Leave the sutures in place until they dissolve and fall out.

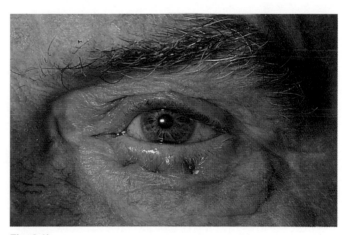

Fig. 6.1b

Complications and management

Overcorrection occurs if the sutures are placed too far down in the fornix or emerge too close to the lashes and are tied too tightly. If ectropion persists for more than a week one or more sutures should be removed.

6:2 Wies

6.2a

Mark the skin incision 4 mm inferior to the lashes medially, 5 mm laterally, and incise the skin. With a lid guard in place make a stab incision through the full thickness of the lid at each end of the incision.

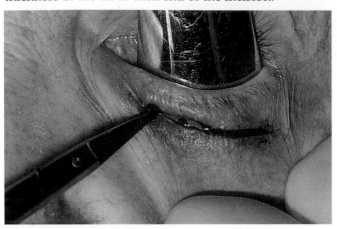

Fig. 6.2a

6.2b

Pass one blade of sharp pointed scissors through both stab incisions and complete the full thickness transverse incision.

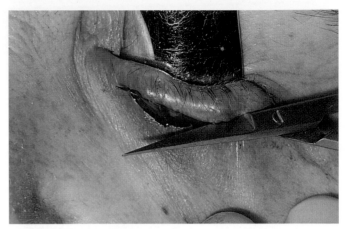

Fig. 6.2b

6.2e

Pass the sutures into the orbicularis muscle anterior to the tarsal plate (arrow) in the upper wound edge to emerge in the skin 2 mm inferior to the lashes.

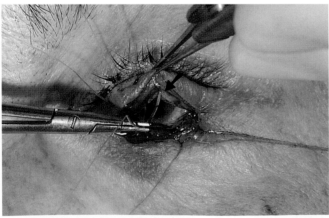

Fig. 6.2e

6.2f

Tie the sutures to achieve a slight ectropion of the lid. Close the skin with a 6/0 suture. Remove the skin sutures at 5 days and the everting sutures at 10 days, or earlier if there is a marked overcorrection.

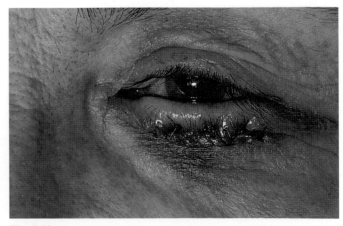

Fig. 6.2f

6.2c

Inspect the lower edge of the incision. The layers from posterior to anterior are conjunctiva, lower lid retractors – which are seen as a white sheet of tissue, usually easily identified – orbicularis and skin.

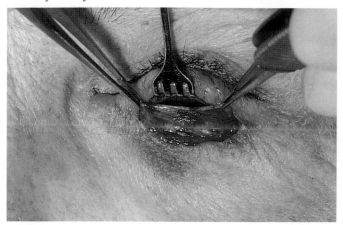

Fig. 6.2c

6.2d

Place three double-armed 4/0 absorbable sutures through the conjunctiva and lower lid retractor layer, 2mm below the cut edge.

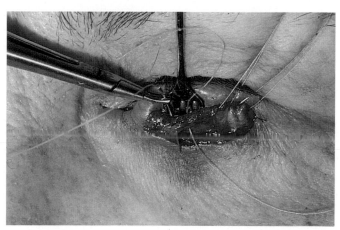

Fig. 6.2d

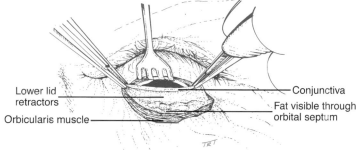

Lower lid retractors
Orbicularis muscle
Conjunctiva
Fat visible through orbital septum

Key diag. 6.2c

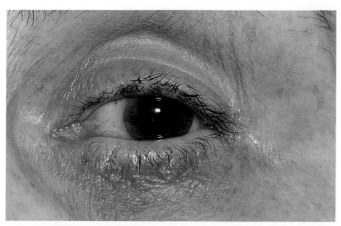

Fig. 6.2 post

Complications and management

Overcorrection may occur if the everting sutures are inserted too far down in the fornix or emerge too close to the lashes. It is also more likely if significant horizontal lid laxity has not been recognised. If overcorrection persists for more than a week remove one or more sutures. If there is no improvement assess horizontal laxity and consider lid shortening (see 2.6).

6:3 **Quickert**

6.3a

Using scissors make a cut 5–6mm long at right angles to the lid margin 5mm medial to the lateral canthus. From the lower end of this cut make a horizontal incision medially, parallel to the lid margin as far as the inferior punctum and 4–5mm from the lid margin. Extend the incision directly laterally (without following the curve of the lid margin) as far as the lateral canthus.

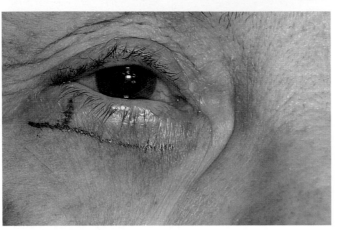

Fig. 6.3a

6.3b

Overlap the marginal strips to estimate how much to excise to correct the horizontal laxity.

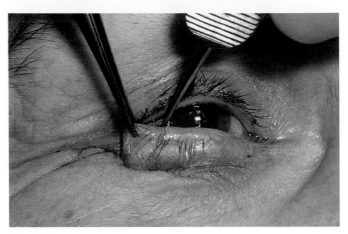

Fig. 6.3b

6.3e

Close the lid margin in the usual way (see 2.6). Tie the sutures to achieve a slight ectropion of the lid. If necessary, a small triangle of skin may be excised laterally (arrow) to avoid a dog-ear in the lower wound edge.

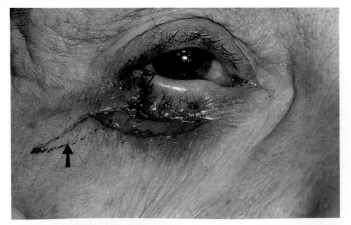

Fig. 6.3e

6.3f

Close the skin with 6/0 sutures.

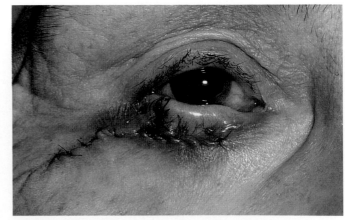

Fig 6.3f

6.3c

Inspect the lower edge of the horizontal incision, identify the lower lid retractors and place three double-armed 4/0 sutures through the conjunctiva and lower lid retractors as described above (6.2d).

6.3d

Pass the three double-armed sutures through orbicularis and skin to emerge 2mm below the lashes as described above (6.2e).

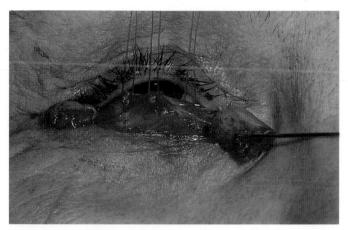

Fig. 6.3c

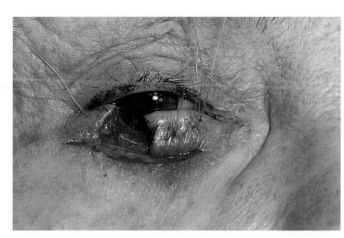

Fig. 6.3d

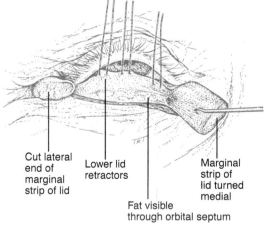

Cut lateral end of marginal strip of lid   Lower lid retractors   Marginal strip of lid turned medial

Fat visible through orbital septum

Key diag. 6.3c

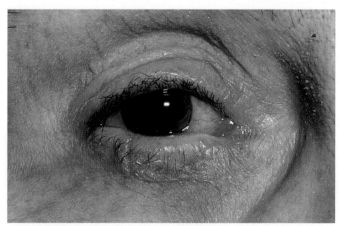

Fig. 6.3 post

Remove the skin sutures at 5 days and the everting sutures at 10 days.

Complications and management

As for the Wies procedure.

6:4 | **Jones**

6.4a

Make an incision through the skin from the punctum to the lateral canthus and 4mm below the lashes. Deepen the incision by separating the bands of orbicularis muscle until the lower border of the tarsal plate is exposed throughout its length. Inspect the lower edge of the incision. Immediately posterior to the (preseptal) orbicularis muscle is the orbital septum which is attached to the lower lid retractors close to the inferior border of the tarsal plate.

6.4b

Carefully dissect or sweep down the skin and muscle layer to expose the septum which can be identified by the fat pad posterior to it.

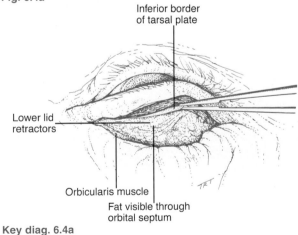

Fig. 6.4a

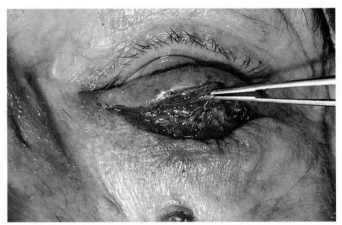

Fig. 6.4b

Inferior border
of tarsal plate

Lower lid
retractors

Orbicularis muscle

Fat visible through
orbital septum

Key diag. 6.4a

6.4c

Incise the septum transversely 2–3 mm below the inferior border of the tarsal plate and retract it and the fat downwards. The white sheet of tissue now visible is the lower lid retractor layer. It moves down with downgaze. The upper border of this layer should be attached to the inferior border of the tarsal plate but it may be detached and is then found a few millimetres inferiorly. When this occurs the conjunctiva is the only layer bridging the gap between the tarsal plate and the lower lid retractors. If the retractors are obviously detached simple reattachment to the inferior border of the tarsal plate with interrupted 6/0 catgut sutures may be all that is needed to stabilise the tarsal plate.

6.4d

If the retractors are found to be attached they will need to be tightened by plication. Pass a 4/0 suture through the centre of the lower skin edge, through the lower lid retractors 8 mm inferior to the tarsus, through the inferior border of the tarsal plate (arrow) and out through the upper skin edge. Tie with a temporary knot and ask the patient to look up and down and observe the effect. If the lid moves normally place two or more similar sutures medial and lateral to the central suture. If, however, the plication is too tight or too loose adjust the position of the lower bite in the lower lid retractors until the correct tension is achieved.

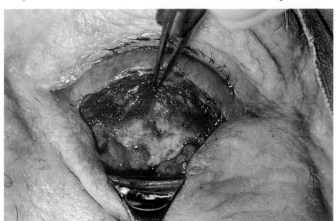

Fig. 6.4c

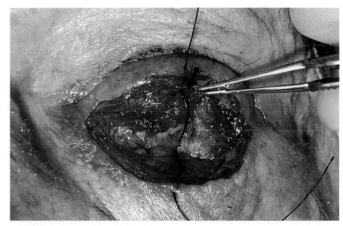

Fig. 6.4d

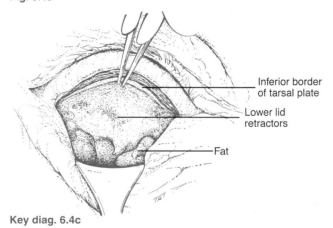

Inferior border of tarsal plate

Lower lid retractors

Fat

Key diag. 6.4c

Technique continues overleaf →

6:4 **Jones** *(Continued)*

6.4e

When all the plicating sutures are in place tie them to close the incision.

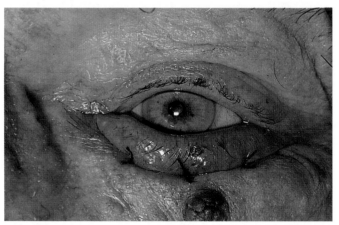

Fig. 6.4e

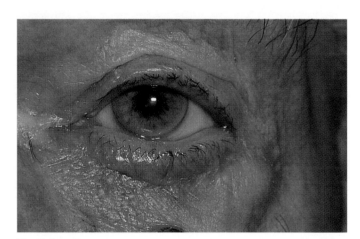

Fig. 6.4 post

Complications and management

Overcorrection or marked retraction of the lower lid margin which persists for more than a week requires removal of one or more of the plicating sutures. Check also that there is no significant horizontal laxity requiring correction.

Cicatricial entropion

Choice of operation

Cicatricial entropion is due to contraction of the posterior lid lamella. Severe cicatricial changes also cause retraction of the whole lid and this must be corrected at the same time as the entropion correction.

In the lower lid mild cicatricial entropion is effectively corrected with a tarsal fracture and everting sutures (6.5).

Severe entropion, often with some lid retraction, requires a posterior lamellar graft (6.6).

In the upper lid mild or moderate cicatricial entropion is corrected with an anterior lamellar reposition (6.7), often with recession of the upper lid retractors. In more severe entropion choose a lamellar division (8.2) if the tarsus is not thickened and a tarsal wedge resection if it is (6.8). If there is marked retraction choose a posterior graft (6.10). If there is keratinisation of the posterior lid margin a lid margin rotation (6.11) is needed.

6:5 Tarsal fracture

6.5a

Place a 4/0 stay suture in the tarsal plate close to the centre of the posterior lid margin. Evert the lid over a Desmarres retractor and make a full thickness incision along the middle of the tarsal plate for its whole length.

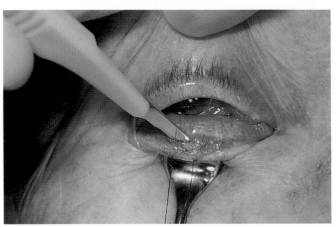

Fig. 6.5a

6.5b

Deepen the incision through the full thickness of the tarsal plate to expose the posterior surface of the pretarsal muscle (arrow). Pass three double-armed 4/0 catgut sutures through the conjunctiva and lower lid retractor layer, attached to the proximal strip of tarsus in the inferior wound edge.

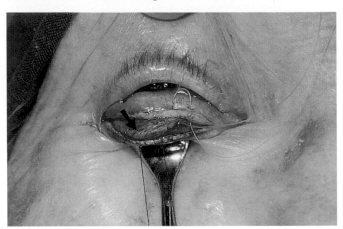

Fig. 6.5b

6.5d

Tie the sutures to overcorrect the entropion. Remove them at 14 days.

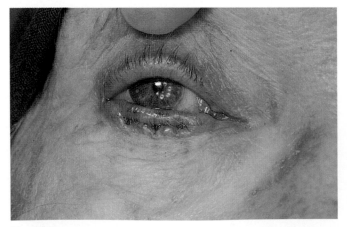

Fig. 6.5d

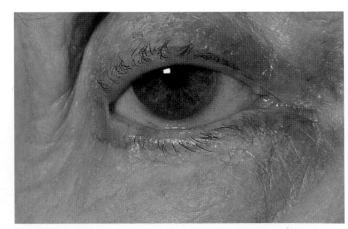

Fig. 6.5 post

Tarsal fracture

6.5c

Pass the sutures through the tissues anterior to the distal strip of tarsus to emerge 1–2 mm below the lashes.

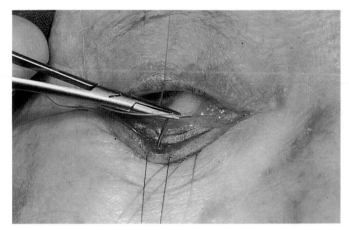

Fig. 6.5c

6:6 Posterior graft (lower lid)

6.6a

Evert the lid over a Desmarres retractor and make a full thickness incision in the tarsal plate as described above (6.5a).

6.6b

Inspect the lower edge of the incision and, dissecting anterior to the lower strip of tarsus, separate the orbicularis muscle anteriorly from the tarsus and septum posteriorly to allow the lower strip of tarsus and the attached septum, lower lid retractors and conjunctiva to fall inferiorly. Take a spacer (see Ch. 2, Sect. D) of sufficient size to fill the gap between the cut edges of the tarsal plate and suture it in place with continuous 6/0 catgut.

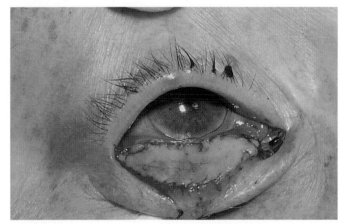

Fig. 6.6b

6.6c

Pass three transverse double-armed 4/0 catgut sutures from the centre of the spacer through the lid obliquely upwards to emerge 1–2 mm below the lashes. Tie the sutures to overcorrect the entropion. Remove them at 7 days.

Complications and management

If a marked overcorrection persists for more than a week remove one or more of the everting sutures.

Complications and management

There is often some irritation of the eye for a week or two. If there is marked overcorrection which persists for more than a week remove one or more of the everting sutures.

6:7 **Anterior lamellar reposition with or without lid split (upper lid)**

6.7a

Make an incision in the skin crease and deepen it through the orbicularis muscle to expose the upper part of the tarsal plate throughout its width. Dissect downwards towards the lashes between the tarsal plate and the orbicularis until the lashes begin to come into view. The anterior and posterior lamellae of the lid have now been separated inferior to the incision. Pull up the anterior lamella in relation to the posterior lamella and assess the amount of correction of the entropion (6.7c).

6.7b

If it is inadequate make an incision along the length of the grey line and deepen it to 2 mm. This allows extra eversion of the lashes when the anterior lamella is sutured.

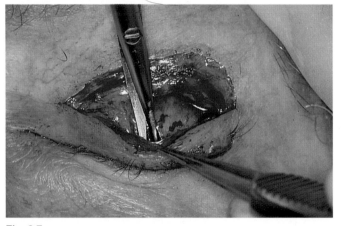

Fig. 6.7a

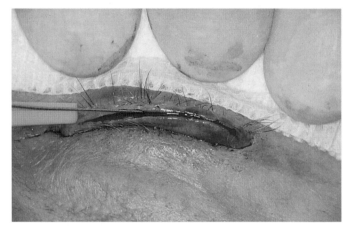

Fig. 6.7b

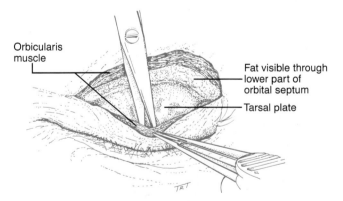

Orbicularis muscle

Fat visible through lower part of orbital septum

Tarsal plate

Key diag. 6.7a

Anterior lamellar reposition with or without lid split (upper lid)

Pull up the anterior lamella again to confirm adequate eversion of the lashes.

Pass three or four 6/0 long-acting absorbable sutures from the skin and orbicularis muscle 1–2 mm above the lashes, through the tarsal plate (arrow) at a level 3–4 mm superiorly and back through the orbicularis and skin 1–2 mm above the lashes.

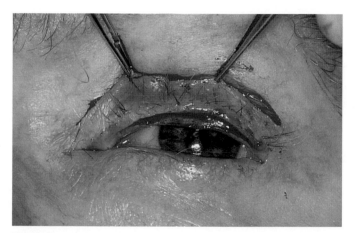

Fig. 6.7c

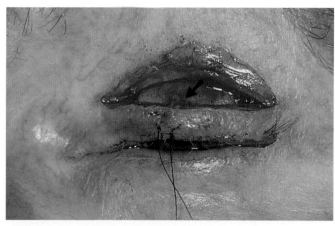

Fig. 6.7d

Tie the sutures to draw the anterior lamella superiorly in relation to the posterior lamella and to evert the lashes. Aim for an overcorrection.

Except in relatively mild degrees of cicatricial entropion retraction of the upper lid may also be present. The upper lid retractors must be recessed to overcome this secondary effect of scarring in the posterior lamella (see 11.3). The septum (arrow) may be opened to confirm the anatomy. To identify it make it bulge by pressure on the lower lid.

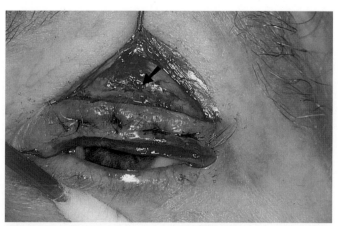

Fig. 6.7e

Technique continues overleaf ➔

6:7   **Anterior lamellar reposition with or without lid split (upper lid)** *(Continued)*

6.7f

Excise a small strip of skin equal in width to the amount of elevation of the anterior lamella. Close the incision with interrupted 6/0 catgut sutures which pick up the anterior surface of the levator aponeurosis (see 9.2h). All the sutures can be left to fall out.

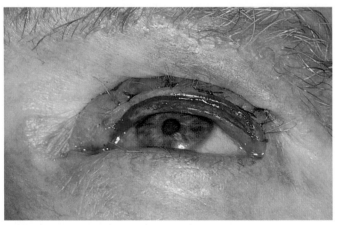

Fig. 6.7f

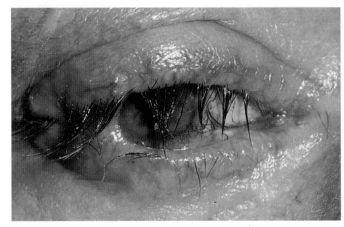

Fig. 6.7 pre

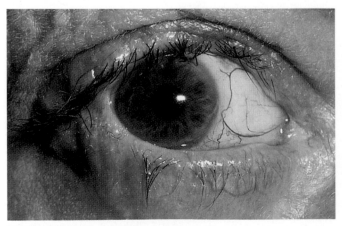

Fig. 6.7 post

Complications and management

If the correction is inadequate wait 6 months and repeat the procedure with a lid split.

6:8 Tarsal wedge resection

This variation of an anterior lamellar reposition is used if the tarsal plate is thick.

6.8a

Expose the tarsal plate, dissect the anterior lamella free and make an incision in the grey line as described above (6.7a–c).

Upper lid retractors recessed

Wedge cut in tarsal plate

Lid margin split

Diag. 6.1

6.8b

Cut out a partial thickness transverse wedge from the middle of the tarsal plate with a blade. To close the wedge in the tarsal plate and evert the lashes place three or four 6/0 long-acting absorbable sutures which pass through the skin and orbicularis muscle 1–2 mm above the lashes, through the tarsal plate just above the wedge, through the tarsal plate just below the wedge, again through the tarsal plate just above the wedge and back through the orbicularis and skin 1–2 mm above the lashes.

6.8c

Recess the upper lid retractors (see 11.3).

From the lower edge of the wound excise a strip of skin equal in width to the amount of elevation of the anterior lamella. Close the incision with 6/0 absorbable sutures which pick up the levator aponeurosis. All sutures may be left to fall out.

6:9 Lamellar division and mucous membrane graft

The technique for this procedure is described and illustrated in 8.2. The exposed tarsal plate may be allowed to granulate or it may be covered with a well-thinned mucous membrane graft (see 2.14) sutured in place with interrupted 6/0 catgut sutures.

Complications and management

Persistent granulations at the lid margin which do not heal may need to be trimmed. Inadequate release of the upper lid retractors may result in lid retraction and the need for further recession (see Ch. 11).

6:10   Posterior graft (upper lid)

Make a full thickness, transverse incision in the middle
of the scarred tarsus. Dissect downwards to allow the
distal tarsal fragment to rotate at the lid margin. Recess
the upper lid retractors (see 11.2). Suture a graft, such
as contralateral tarsal plate (see 2.17) or oral mucous
membrane (see 2.13), into the space between the
separated edges of the scarred tarsus. Use buried
absorbable sutures at the upper edge. Halfway, insert
sutures to fix the graft and support the anterior lamella
in its recessed position. At the lower edge pass sutures
from the skin into the graft and tie them on the skin to
hold the lid margin everted.

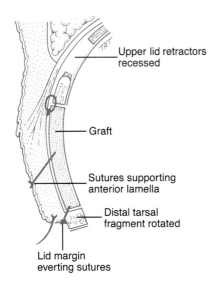

Diag. 6.2

6:11   Lid margin rotation (Trabut)

6.11a

Evert the lid and, ideally, hold it in place with a
Crookshank or Barrie Jones clamp. Incise the full
thickness of the tarsal plate transversely just superior
to the strip of keratinisation.

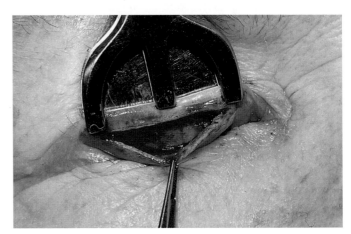

Fig. 6.11a

6.11b

Turn the tarsal plate down and dissect superiorly along its anterior surface to separate the orbicularis muscle from the tarsal plate and orbital septum. Identify the superior border of the tarsal plate and separate off the upper lid retractors and any fibrosis. Continue the dissection upwards posterior to Muller's muscle as far as the fornix trying to preserve the conjunctiva. The tarsal plate should now move freely down in relation to the anterior lamella of the lid.

6.11c

Undermine the distal strip of tarsus (arrow) to separate it from the orbicularis muscle almost to the lid margin. Make a small relieving incision through the strip of tarsus at the lateral canthus and another just lateral to the punctum so that it can be freely rotated through 180 degrees.

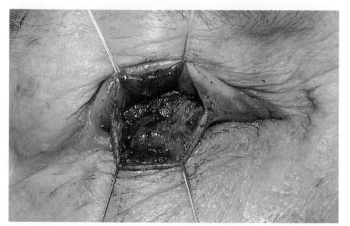

Fig. 6.11b

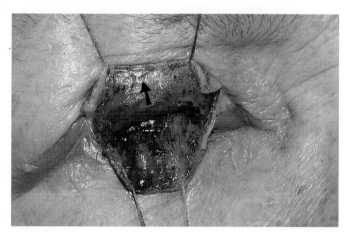

Fig. 6.11c

Keratinised posterior
lid margin

Sutures in
orbicularis muscle

Upper lid retractors
Freed from tarsal
plate

Conjunctiva
Tarsal plate

Cut edge of
tarsal plate

Key diag. 6.11b

Technique continues overleaf ➔

6:11 Lid margin rotation (Trabut) *(Continued)*

6.11d

Pass three double-armed 4/0 catgut sutures obliquely down through the lid from the conjunctiva just above the tarsal plate to the skin crease and tie them over small cotton wool bolsters (as in 9.3i) to hold the anterior lamella in a recessed position. The cut edge of the rotated strip of tarsus should be level with the cut edge of the main tarsal plate (arrow). Suture the two together with interrupted 6/0 Dexon or Vicryl sutures tied on the anterior surface.

6.11e

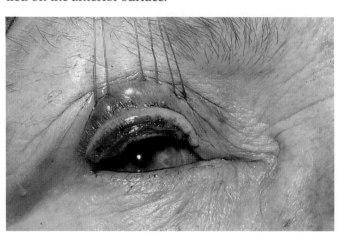

Fig. 6.11d

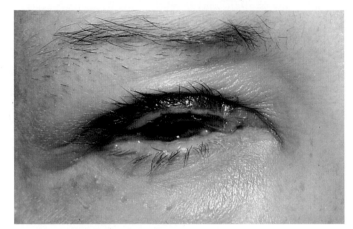

Fig. 6.11 post (different case)

Complications and management

The lid margin takes several weeks to heal fully. Inadequate eyelid closure requires further recession of the upper lid retractors.

Alternative procedures

6:12 Excision of the tarsal plate

A severely scarred, contracted upper lid tarsus may rarely have to be excised completely to achieve a satisfactory position of the lid margin. An alternative procedure should be used if possible to avoid complete excision of the tarsus which creates instability of the lid.

Excision of the tarsal plate

The lid is split into anterior and posterior lamellae and the tarsus is excised. Dissect superiorly between Muller's muscle and the levator muscle to achieve comfortable lid closure. Recess the levator further if necessary. Pass three double-armed catgut sutures through the lid from the edge of the recessed conjunctiva and retractors to the skin at the skin crease.

Congenital entropion

Choice of operation

Surgical correction is not needed for mild epiblepharon. Severe, symptomatic epiblepharon and true congenital entropion are corrected with excision of a strip of skin and muscle and fixation of the skin crease to the tarsal plate. Bilateral surgery ensures a cosmetic result because of symmetrical scars.

Involutional ectropion

Choice of operation

If the medial canthal tendon is lax stabilise it by attachment to the posterior lacrimal crest (7.4, 7.5).

If the lateral canthal tendon is obviously lax correct it with a lateral canthal sling (7.9).

Correct any residual ectropion with horizontal lid shortening (7.1).

If there is a marked excess of skin in the lower lid this may be excised at the time of the ectropion correction with a Kuhnt–Zymanowski procedure (7.3).

If the ectropion is mainly medial and the medial canthal tendon is intact correct the punctal ectropion and any horizontal laxity with a Lazy-T procedure (7.2).

7:1   Horizontal lid shortening

Plan to excise a pentagon of full thickness eyelid (see 2.6) where the ectropion is most marked. If there is significant laxity of the medial canthal tendon this must be corrected first, before this or any other procedure which tightens the lid.

7.1a

Having made the first incision at right angles to the lid margin at the chosen site, which is often in the lateral third of the lid, overlap the cut edges to estimate the horizontal length of lid to be excised (as in Fig. 7.2a). Aim at good apposition of the lid to the eye but avoid undue tension across the closure.

7.1b

Excise the redundant lid and close in the usual way (see 2.6).

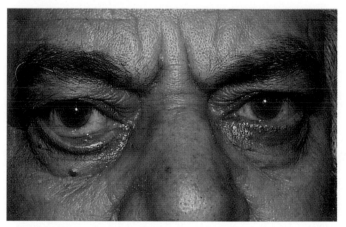

Fig. 7.1 pre

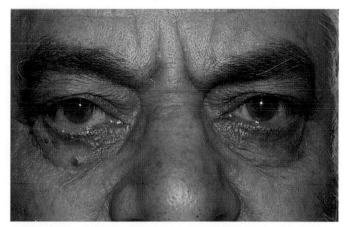

Fig. 7.1 post

Complications and management

If the lower lid retractors are lax or detached tightening the lid may cause the tarsal plate to evert completely. This can be corrected by reattaching the lower lid retractors to the inferior border of the tarsal plate or tucking them with a Jones procedure (see Ch. 6.4).

7:2   Tarsoconjunctival diamond excision with horizontal shortening ('Lazy-T')

7.2a

Make an incision through the full thickness of the lower lid 4mm lateral to the punctum. Overlap the cut edges and excise the excess tissue as a pentagon (see 2.6).

7.2b

Using sharp-pointed scissors and starting at the medial cut edge excise a horizontal diamond of tarsoconjunctiva whose widest point is below the punctum. Leave 2mm between the punctum and the superior edge of the diamond. Pass one needle of a double-armed 6/0 absorbable suture through the conjunctiva immediately below the punctum then obliquely through the lid to the skin at a level about 5mm lower. Pass the other needle through the conjunctiva and lower lid retractors at the opposite edge of the diamond then obliquely through the lid to the skin just below the first needle. When this suture is tied the punctal ectropion will be corrected.

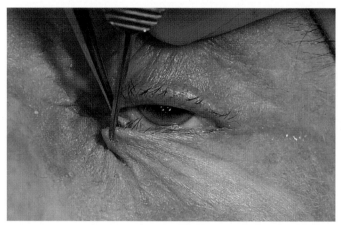

Fig. 7.2a

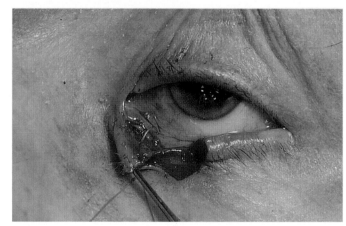

Fig. 7.2b

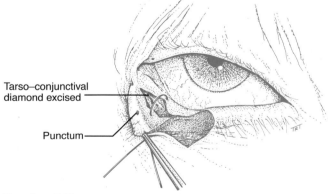

Tarso–conjunctival diamond excised

Punctum

Key diag. 7.2b

Tarsoconjunctival diamond excision with horizontal shortening ('Lazy-T')

7.2c

Tie the inverting suture on the skin – a bolster may be used. Close the lid in the usual way. Remove the sutures in 2 weeks.

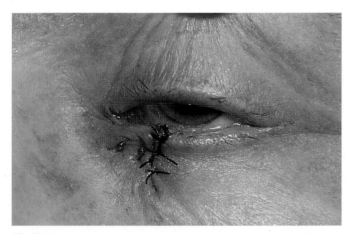

Fig. 7.2c

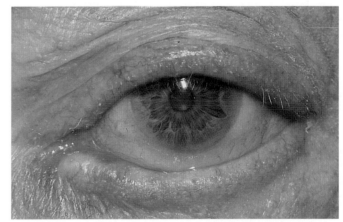

7.2 pre

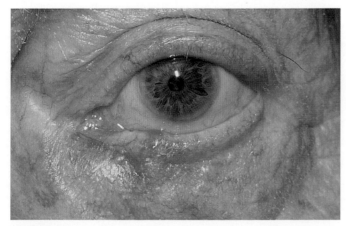

7.2 post

Complications and management

Persistent eversion of the punctum may be due to inadequate excision of posterior lamellar tissue or to distortion of the lid margin at the site of direct closure. Once the lid has healed with a persistently everted punctum retropunctal cautery is often effective.

7:3   Horizontal shortening and blepharoplasty (Kuhnt–Zymanowski)

This technique is similar to a skin flap blepharophlasty of the lower lid (see 10.5).

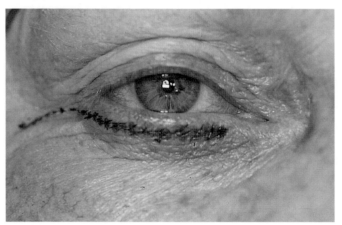

7.3a

Mark the skin incision 2 mm below the lashes from the inferior punctum to the lateral canthus. Extend this obliquely downwards in a skin crease.

Fig. 7.3a

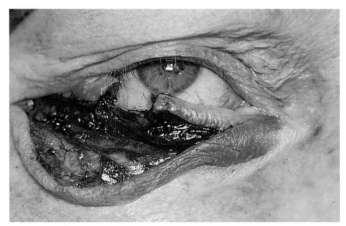

7.3b

Raise the skin flap without orbicularis muscle. Shorten the lid as described in 7.1 above.

Fig. 7.3b

7.3e

Excise the lateral triangle of redundant skin. Close the subciliary incision with a continuous 6/0 suture and the skin crease incision with interrupted 6.0 sutures.

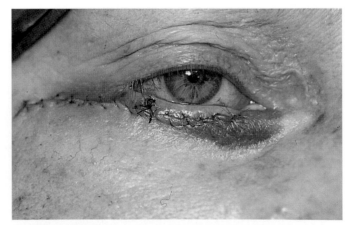

Fig. 7.3e

Horizontal shortening and blepharoplasty (Kuhnt–Zymanowski)

7.3c

Replace the skin flap, drawing it up and laterally but with minimal tension.

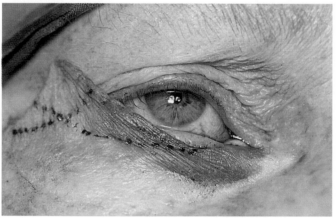

Fig. 7.3c

7.3d

Excise the superior triangle of redundant skin.

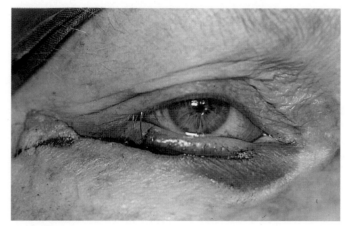

Fig. 7.3d

Complications and management

See 'Horizontal lid shortening' (7.1) and 'Lower lid blepharoplasty' (Ch. 10, Sect. B).

7:4   Stabilisation of medial canthal tendon – conjunctival approach

The tendon must be reattached to the posterior lacrimal crest. This approach is suitable if the laxity is not very marked.

7.4a

Place a probe in the lower lacrimal canaliculus. Make an incision in the conjunctiva just lateral to the plica and extend it inferiorly to expose the medial end of the tarsal plate (arrow).

7.4b

Dissect posteriorly with blunt dissection staying just lateral to the lacrimal sac until the posterior lacrimal crest can be felt. Take care to avoid damage to the medial rectus muscle. Spread the tissues gently and insert malleable retractors to expose the posterior lacrimal crest with its periosteum intact (arrow). Pass both needles of a 5/0 double-armed suture through the periosteum of the posterior lacrimal crest at the level of the medial canthus.

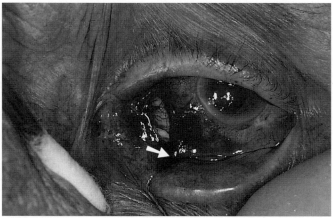

Fig. 7.4a

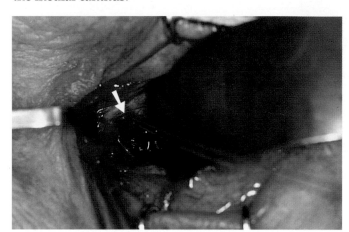

Fig. 7.4b

7.4e

Tighten the 5/0 suture, tying it anteriorly, and bury the knot in the orbicularis muscle. Ensure a satisfactory position of the lid before tying.

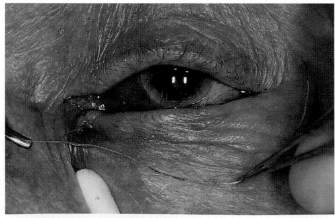

Fig. 7.4e

Stabilisation of medial canthal tendon – conjunctival approach

7.4c

Make a horizontal skin incision 2mm inferior to the punctum to expose the medial end of the tarsal plate. Pass the needles through the medial end of the lower tarsal plate under direct vision and as close to the lid margin as possible. Some adjustment of the position of the sutures in the tarsal plate is frequently necessary to achieve a good position of the medial end of the lid when the sutures are tightened and tied.

7.4d

Before tightening the 5/0 suture close the conjunctiva to cover this suture (arrow) – the edges may be difficult to locate once the canthal tendon is tight.

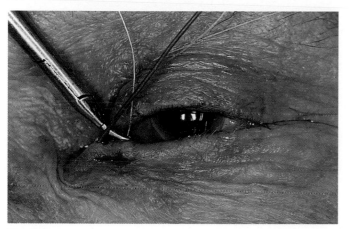

Fig. 7.4c

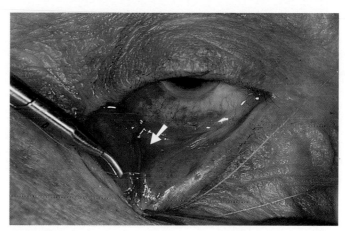

Fig. 7.4d

7.4f

Close the skin incision with interrupted 6/0 non-absorbable sutures.

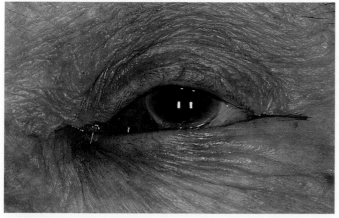

Fig. 7.4f

Complications and management

Conjunctival chemosis is common at the inner canthus and may persist for several weeks postoperatively. Eversion of the inferior punctum and distortion of the lid may arise because of difficulty with the placement of the suture in the tarsal plate. If distortion occurs allow the lid to heal. The distortion reduces with time and if it is still unsatisfactory at 6 months a medial wedge excision (7.5) will be necessary to correct it.

7:5   Medial wedge excision

This approach is suitable if the canthal tendon laxity is very marked as, for example, in a long standing facial palsy.

7.5a

Make a vertical cut through the full thickness of the lid 3–4mm lateral to the medial canthus, medial to the punctum.

7.5b

Gently pull the lateral cut edge of the lid medially and resect the excess as a pentagon. Aim at correction of the horizontal laxity without undue tension.

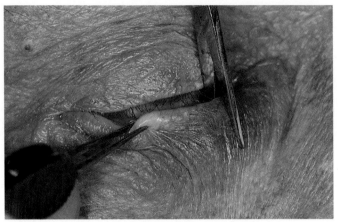

Fig. 7.5a

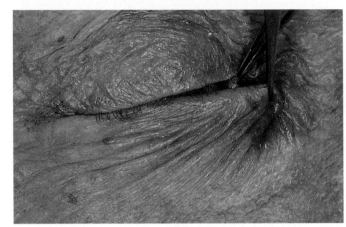

Fig. 7.5b

7.5e

Cut the canaliculus longitudinally for 3–4 mm.

7.5f

Separate the cut edges of the opened canaliculus and place two 7/0 absorbable sutures between the corners and the adjacent conjunctiva. This will help to hold the canaliculus open.

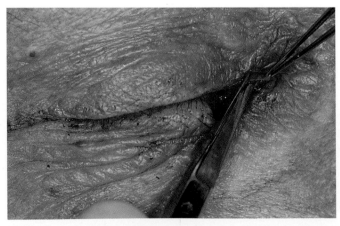

Fig. 7.5e

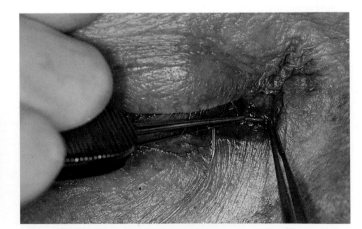

Fig. 7.5f

7.5c

Identify the lower canaliculus (arrow) in the medial cut edge. Place a probe in the canaliculus (removed for the photograph). Using blunt dissection with scissors directed posteriorly and medially, lateral to the lacrimal sac, palpate and expose the posterior lacrimal crest at or just above the level of the medial canthus.

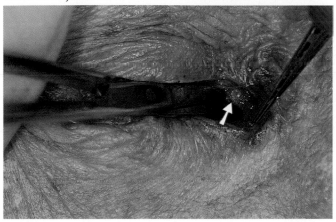

Fig. 7.5c

7.5d

Place a malleable retractor to improve the exposure and insert both needles of a double-armed 5/0 non-absorbable suture, directed posteriorly through the periosteum of the posterior lacrimal crest (arrow).

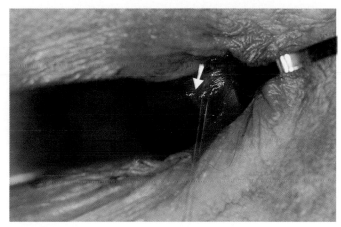

Fig. 7.5d

7.5g

Pass one needle of the 5/0 suture through the tarsal plate close to the lid margin, adjusting its position as necessary so that when the suture is tightened the lid is drawn medially and posteriorly to lie against the eye.

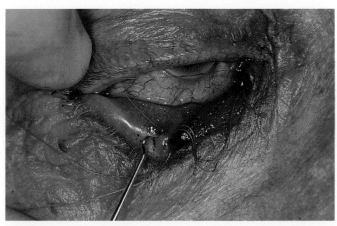

Fig. 7.5g

Pass the second needle through the tarsal plate 2–3 mm inferior to the first. Pass a 7/0 absorbable suture through the lip of the canaliculus and through the conjunctiva of the lateral cut edge.

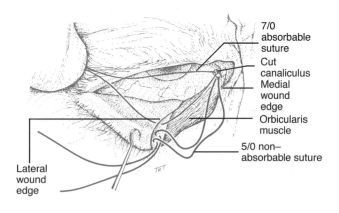

7/0 absorbable suture
Cut canaliculus
Medial wound edge
Orbicularis muscle
5/0 non–absorbable suture
Lateral wound edge

Key diag. 7.5g

Technique continues overleaf ➜

7:5 **Medial wedge excision** *(Continued)*

7.5h

Tie the 5/0 suture with a single throw to draw the lateral wound edge medially. Tie the 7/0 suture (arrow) to marsupialise the canaliculus into the conjunctival sac.

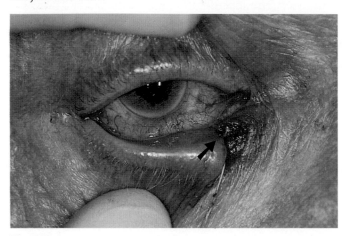

Fig. 7.5h

7.5i

Close the conjunctiva to ensure that the 5/0 fixation suture is well covered. Tighten the 5/0 fixation suture further and tie it.

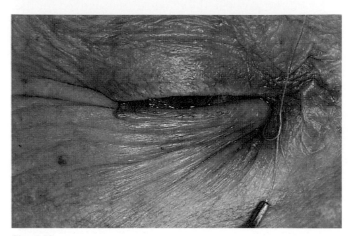

Fig. 7.5i

7.5j

Close the skin with 6/0 sutures.

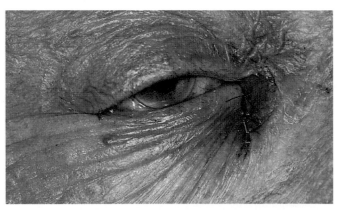

Fig. 7.5j

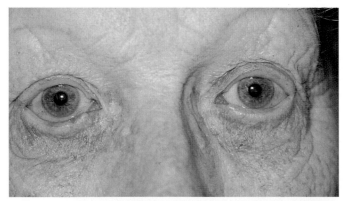

7.5 pre

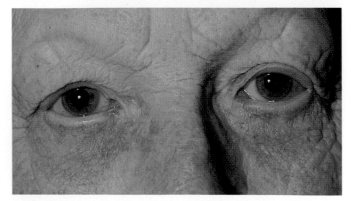

7.5 post

Complications and management

The medial end of the lid may be held away from the eye – this follows if the fixation suture is not placed posteriorly enough. Local oedema may contribute immediately postoperatively. Wait until the lid is healed and if the unsatisfactory position persists reopen the wound at 6 months and reattach the lid to the posterior lacrimal crest.

Cicatricial ectropion

Choice of operation

Use a Z-plasty (7.6 and see 2.20) to correct shortening due to a linear scar and insert a full thickness skin graft (7.7 and see Ch. 2, Sect. C) to correct a generalised contraction of lower lid skin.

7:6 **Z-plasty (see 2.20)**

7.6a

Mark the edges of the linear scar.

7.6b

If the scar is causing a notch at the lid margin excise a pentagon of lid to include the upper part of the scar as far as the inferior border of the tarsal plate. Close the lid margin in the usual way. Excise the remaining scar.

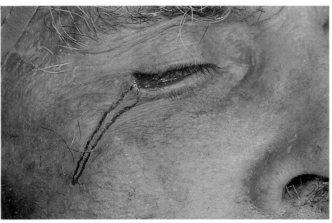

Fig. 7.6a

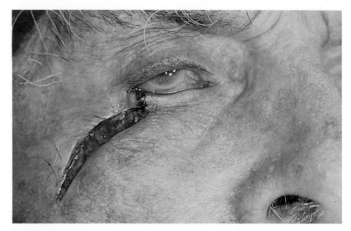

Fig. 7.6b

7.6d

Reflect the skin flaps and undermine the skin well beyond the limits of the flaps. Excise any deeper residual scar tissue. Transpose the flaps (see 2.20) and suture with 6/0 sutures. Place a traction suture at the lid margin and maintain upward traction on the lid for 48 hours.

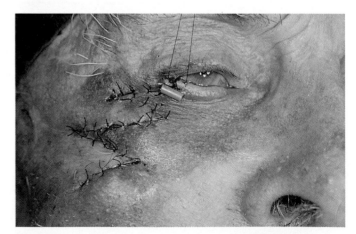

Fig. 7.6d

7.6c

From each end of the linear defect mark lines at 60 degrees and equal in length to the defect to fashion the Z. Two or more Zs can be marked along longer scars, as in the case illustrated.

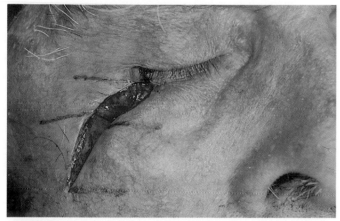

Fig. 7.6c

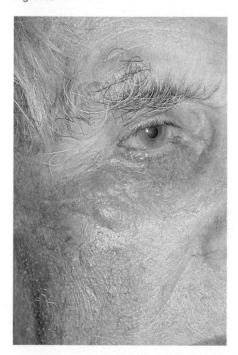

7.6 post

Complications and management

See 2.20. Persistent ectropion is usually due to inadequate lengthening of the scar. A small skin graft may be needed to correct it.

7:7 Skin graft

A graft of full thickness skin (see Ch. 2, Sect. C) is preferable to split thickness skin to correct a diffuse scar in the lower lid.

7.7a

Mark the incision 2–3 mm below the lid margin extending for several millimetres either side of the contracted area.

7.7b

Undermine the contracted skin until the ectropion of the lid margin is fully corrected.

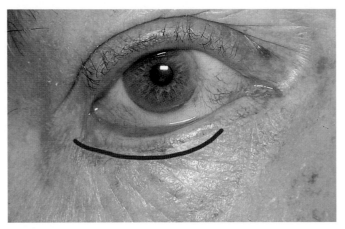

Fig. 7.7a

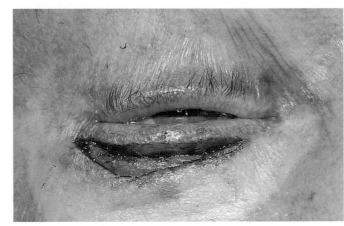

Fig. 7.7b

7.7A–C

Much larger grafts are often needed.

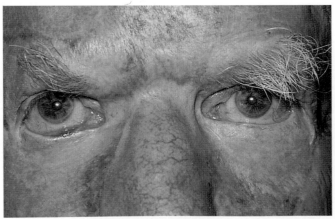

7.7A

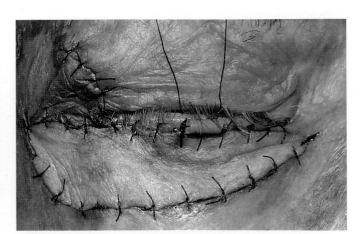

7.7B

7.7c

If there is significant horizontal lid laxity shorten the lid (arrow) (see 7.1). Place one or two lid margin sutures through the grey line to provide traction. Take a full thickness skin graft from the upper lid or from behind the ear as described in Chapter 2, Section C. Suture the graft into the defect maintaining gentle traction on the lid margin. If a flavine wool tie-over bolster is to be used leave alternate sutures long (see Ch. 2, Sect. C).

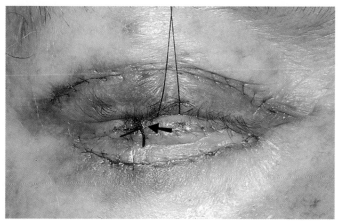

Fig. 7.7c

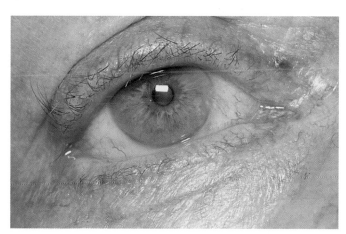

7.7 post

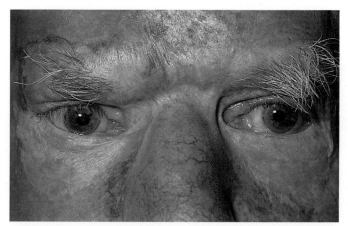

7.7C

Complications and management

See Chapter 2, Section C.

Incomplete correction of the ectropion is due either to persistent horizontal lid laxity or too small a graft. Wait for 6 months if possible before further surgery.

Paralytic ectropion

Choice of operation

Correct medial ectropion first with a medial wedge excision (7.5) if the medial canthal tendon is lax or a medial canthoplasty (7.8) if the medial canthal tendon is intact. Correct residual ectropion by tightening the lid with a lateral canthal sling (7.9).

7:9   Lateral ca

7:8   Medial canthoplasty

7.9a

Make a horizontal inci
the lateral orbit rim (a
through the orbicularis

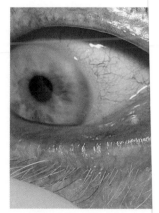

Fig. 7.9a

7.9c

Pull the cut tendon later
orbital septum on stretcl
subconjunctivally along
the lateral one-third of tl
move laterally more free

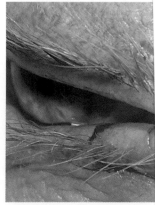

Fig. 7.9c

7.8a

Place lacrimal probes in the canaliculi. Make incisions along the lid margins from the puncta to the inner canthus leaving the canaliculi in the posterior lamellae.

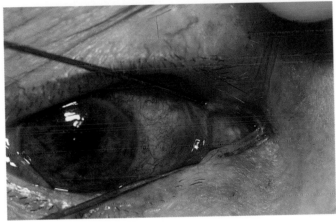

Fig. 7.8a

7.8b

Undermine the skin to expose the orbicularis muscle beyond the canaliculi above and below. Place one or two 6/0 absorbable sutures which pass from the muscle above the upper canaliculus to the muscle below the lower canaliculus.

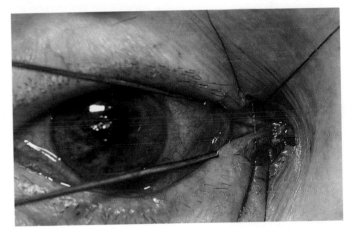

Fig. 7.8b

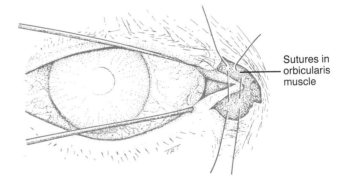

Sutures in orbicularis muscle

Key diag 7.8b

Technique continues overleaf →

7:8 | Media

7:9 | **Lateral canthal sling** *(Continued)*

7.9e

Trim the lower border of the tarsal plate to elongate the lateral canthal tendon in a medial direction.

7.9f

Pass this refashioned lower limb of the lateral canthal tendon through a buttonhole in the upper limb of the tendon, or posterior to it, and attach the lower limb to the periosteum of the lateral orbital rim with a 5/0 non-absorbable suture. It should be under sufficient tension to correct the horizontal laxity in the lid.

7.8c

Tie the sutures to
lacrimal puncta a

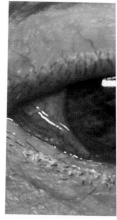

Fig. 7.8c

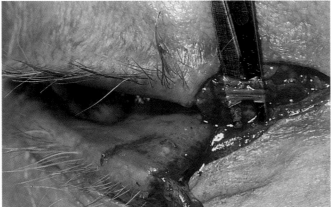

Fig. 7.9e

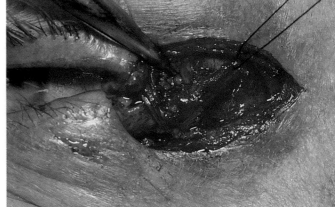

Fig. 7.9f

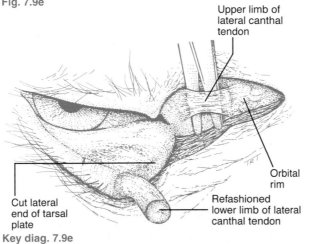

Upper limb of
lateral canthal
tendon

Orbital
rim

Cut lateral
end of tarsal
plate

Refashioned
lower limb of lateral
canthal tendon

Key diag. 7.9e

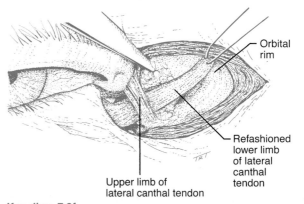

Orbital
rim

Refashioned
lower limb
of lateral
canthal
tendon

Upper limb of
lateral canthal tendon

Key diag. 7.9f

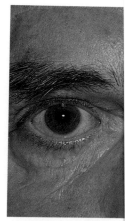

7.8 post

7.9g

Close the incision in two layers with 6/0 sutures.

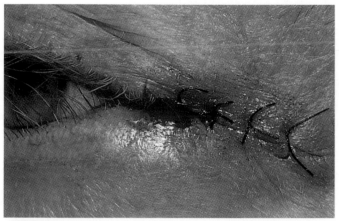

Fig. 7.9g

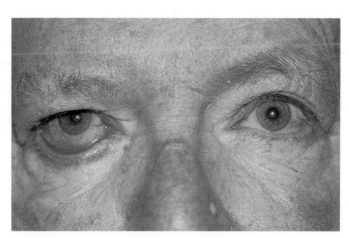

7.9 pre

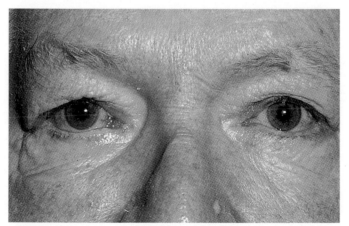

7.9 post A

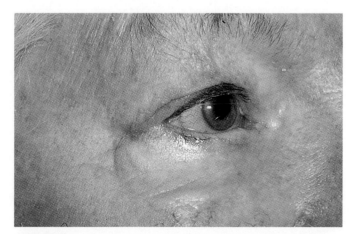

7.9 post B

Complications and management

Overlapping lids at the lateral canthus can be avoided by careful approximation of the lid margins at the lateral canthus.

Alternative procedures

7:10 **Medial canthal tendon plication**	**7:11** **Autogenous fascia lata sling**

Through an incision close to the lid margin medial to the lower punctum identify the anterior limb of the medial canthal tendon. Suture the tarsal plate to the medial remnant of canthal tendon with a 5/0 non-absorbable suture.

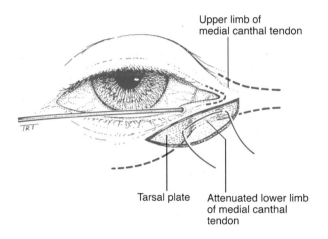

Upper limb of
medial canthal tendon

Tarsal plate   Attenuated lower limb
of medial canthal
tendon

Diag. 7.1

This procedure often causes the medial end of the lid to be drawn away from the eye. This effect can be mini-mised by tightening the suture just enough to stabilise the canthal tendon. Reattachment of the lid to the posterior lacrimal crest is usually preferable (see 7.4, 7.5).

Take a narrow strip of fascia lata in the usual way (see 2.18). Expose the medial canthal tendon through a vertical incision 8 mm medial to the inner canthus. Expose the lateral orbital rim through a vertical incision and drill two holes through the rim having reflected the periosteum. Using a Wright's fascia lata needle, or equivalent, insert a strip of fascia lata 2 mm wide deep to the orbicularis muscle, close to the lash line, between the medial and lateral incisions. Loop it around the medial canthal tendon to fix it medially and, having tightened it to support the lid, pass it through the holes in the lateral orbital rim. Make an incision over the band in the centre of the lid and suture it to the tarsal plate.

This technique is useful particularly with an anophthalmic socket to support an artificial eye.

RELATED DISORDERS

Management of facial palsy

a) Acute phase and first 3 months –
   recovery possible
   — diagnosis of the cause
   — corneal protection with simple and
     reversible treatment:
     — lubricants
     — temporary tarsorrhaphy (11.8)

b) Assessment at 3 months
   — no recovery: ?nerve grafting or
     anastomosis planned
     — medial canthoplasty (7.8)
     — lateral canthal sling (7.9)
   — partial recovery:
     — wait

c) Assessment at 6 months and after
   — incomplete recovery:
     — medial wedge excision (7.5)
     — brow fixation (10.7)
     — Muller's muscle excision (11.1)
     — ? Jones' tube

Management of burns of the eyelids

a) Partial thickness: lid retraction and
   corneal exposure usually mild
   — wait, topical lubricants
   — split skin graft if necessary

b) Full thickness:
   — lid retraction and corneal exposure
     often severe, topical lubricants alone
     usually inadequate
   — remove dead tissue; large split skin
     graft (see Ch. 2, Sect. C) extending
     beyond the medial and lateral canthi.
     Use dental moulding material (e.g.
     Stent), or moist cotton wool, as a
     bolster, secured with sutures. Grafting
     may need to be repeated if further
     contraction occurs.

FURTHER READING

Anderson R L, Gordy D D: The tarsal strip procedure. Arch Ophthalmol 97: 2192; 1979

Collin J R O: A manual of systematic eyelid surgery, 2nd edn. Churchill Livingstone, Edinburgh; 1989

Crawford G J, Collin J R O, Moriarty P A J: The correction of paralytic medial ectropion. Br J Ophthalmol 68: 639; 1984

Dutton J J: Surgical management of the floppy eyelid syndrome. Am J Ophthalmol 99: 557; 1985

Lee O S: Operation for correction of everted lacrimal puncta. Am J Ophthalmol 34: 575; 1951

Smith B: The 'Lazy-T' correction of ectropion of the lower punctum. Arch Ophthalmol 94: 1149; 1976

Sullivan T J, Collin J R O: Medial canthal resection: An effective long term cure for medial ectropion. Br J Ophthalmol 75: 288; 1991

Tenzel R R: Treatment of lagophthalmos of the lower lid. Arch Ophthalmol 81: 366; 1969

CHAPTER 8

Eyelash abnormalities

Introduction

Although ingrowing lashes are usually only a minor irritant they may cause permanent scarring of the cornea and threaten sight, especially if the cornea is insensitive or the eye is dry.

Classification: Trichiasis
                                          Distichiasis

Trichiasis is a common, acquired, misdirection of eyelashes arising from their normal site of origin. Distichiasis is a rare, congenital growth of an extra row of eyelashes arising from the meibomian gland orifices. In both, the position of the lid margin is normal. If there is entropion of the lid margin this must be treated first (see Chap. 6) before treatment of the abnormal lashes.

Trichiasis

Choice of operation

Electrolysis is preferred for the treatment of a small number of isolated lashes. Cryotherapy is more effective for many abnormal lashes. If there is a concentration of abnormal lashes in only one site along the lid margin the area may be excised (see Ch. 2.6).

8:1   Cryotherapy

A nitrous oxide probe is preferred to a liquid nitrogen spray for the treatment of lashes because of better control of the temperature and of the area treated. The use of a thermocouple is important until the time taken to reach the required temperature with a particular cryoprobe can be predicted accurately. A double freeze-thaw cycle to −20°C is used.

8.1a

Anaesthetise the lid with 2% lignocaine with 1:200 000 adrenaline.

8.1b

With a corneal guard in place apply the cryoprobe for the appropriate duration (usually 20–30 seconds, depending on the probe used), allow the ice ball to thaw and reapply the cryoprobe for the same duration. Remove the lashes from the area of the cryotherapy.

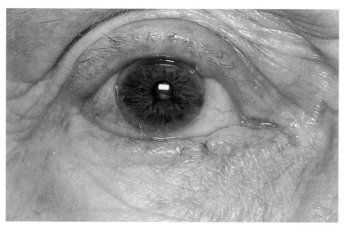

Fig. 8.1a

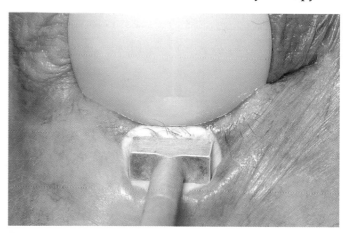

Fig. 8.1b

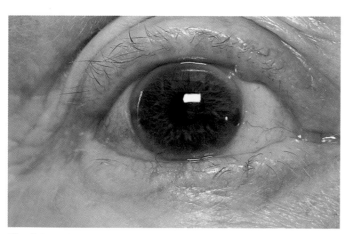

Fig. 8.1 post

Complications and management

Melanocytes are destroyed at −10°C so depigmented patches will appear if this treatment is used on pigmented skin.
Shallow notches and skin sloughing will follow excessive treatment.
Recurrent lashes may be retreated.

Levator aponeurotic repair

Choice of approach to the levator

The anterior (skin) approach is familiar, it allows skin to be excised and it leaves the conjunctiva intact. The posterior (conjunctival) approach although less familiar at first allows more postoperative control of the lid height.

9:2   Anterior levator aponeurotic repair

The upper lid skin crease is usually raised by a levator aponeurotic defect. A new skin crease is made 6–8 mm from the lash line.

9.2a

Mark the skin crease symmetrical with the opposite side or at the desired level in bilateral cases and make an incision through the skin to expose the underlying orbicularis muscle. Lift the skin edges at either side of centre of the wound with fine toothed forceps and deepen the wound through the orbicularis muscle until the tarsal plate is exposed throughout the length of the incision. Take care not to stray down towards the lashes or upwards above the upper tarsal border.

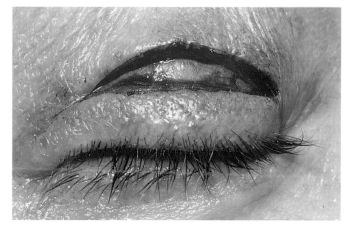

Fig. 9.2a

9.2b

Identify the orbicularis muscle layer in the upper wound edge. Immediately deep to this layer is the white levator aponeurosis, the end of which was probably cut while deepening the first incision. Dissect upwards immediately posterior to the orbicularis for about a centimetre to expose the orbital septum. Take care that this dissection is in the correct plane and not in the deeper, easier plane between the levator aponeurosis and Muller's muscle. When the dissection is in the correct plane the posterior surface of the orbicularis muscle fibres can be seen clearly without any overlying sheet of tissue. It may also be possible to see the whitish-yellow preaponeurotic fat pad through the orbital septum and pressure on the lower eyelid may make the fat pad push the septum forward. Often, however, layers of fine connective tissue overlying the septum mask the presence of the fat pad until they are removed.

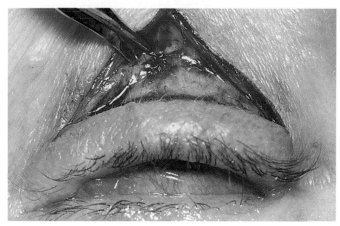

Fig. 9.2b

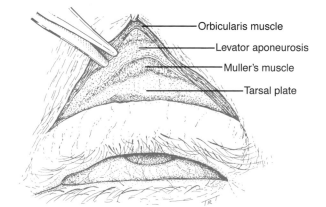

— Orbicularis muscle
— Levator aponeurosis
— Muller's muscle
— Tarsal plate

Key diag. 9.2b

Technique continues overleaf →

9:2 Anterior levator aponeurotic repair *(Continued)*

9.2g

If there is excess skin above the wound mark the skin to be removed and excise it with scissors. Begin the excision with a central vertical cut from the wound edge.

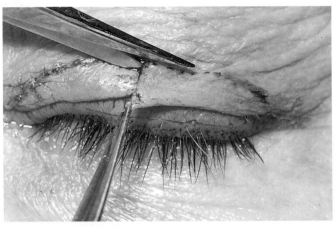

Fig. 9.2g

9.2h

Close the skin with a 6/0 suture taking a bite of the levator aponeurosis (arrow) at the level of the skin crease. Absorbable sutures should be used in children and may be used in adults.

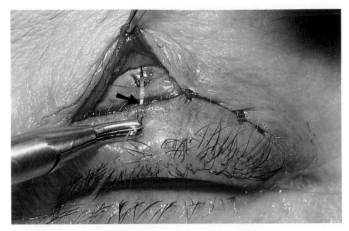

Fig. 9.2h

9.2i

Insert a Frost suture (see 2.19) and tape it to the brow to protect the cornea under the dressing.

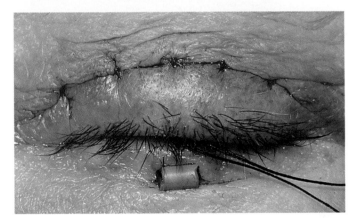

Fig. 9.2i

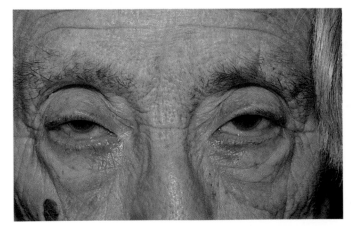

Fig. 9.2 pre

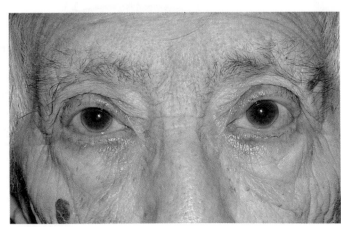

Fig. 9.2 post

9:3   Posterior levator aponeurotic repair

9.3a

Mark the skin crease as in 9.2 above, evert the lid and place a stay suture through the tarsal plate close to the lid margin. Insert a Desmarres retractor and evert the lid over it to stabilise the tarsal plate. Make a short transverse cut through the centre of the tarsal plate close to the superior tarsal border, approximately level with the skin crease. The postaponeurotic space, an easily identified surgical space, will be entered (see Diag. 1.7).

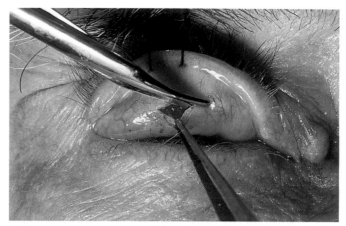

Fig. 9.3a

9.3b

Enlarge the incision in the tarsal plate transversely, parallel to the lid margin, extending it into the conjunctiva medially and laterally. The attenuated levator aponeurosis is the structure visible in the depths of the wound. Dissect upwards between the aponeurosis and Muller's muscle which is inserted into the strip of superior tarsal border (see Diag. 1.7).

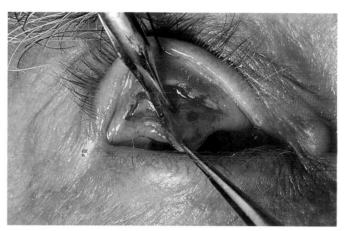

Fig. 9.3b

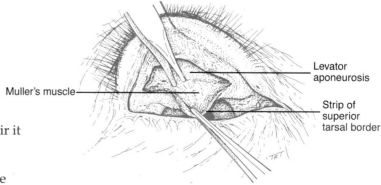

Muller's muscle ⎯⎯⎯

Levator aponeurosis

Strip of superior tarsal border

Key diag. 9.3b

Note – As in an anterior approach aponeurotic repair it is not always essential to open the septum. It can, however, be opened to confirm the anatomy or to identify healthy aponeurosis if it is not found where expected. To do this remove the Desmarres retractor and replace it over the everted tarsal plate and the orbicularis muscle above it. Identify the septum and incise it transversely (see 9.2c, d, 9.5a–c) to expose the preaponeurotic fat pad and the underlying levator muscle with Whitnall's ligament (see 9.7a).

Technique continues overleaf ➔

9:4   **Anterior levator resection** *(Continued)*

9.4k

If a very large levator resection is needed the amount of functioning muscle may be reduced. By placing the levator over Whitnall's ligament the fulcrum of action of the levator is raised and less muscle needs to be resected to achieve the same effect.

Carefully dissect the muscle from beneath Whitnall's ligament. Begin by cutting the muscle sheath transversely above and below Whitnall's.

9.4l

Place the muscle over the ligament. Attach it to the tarsal plate in the usual way.

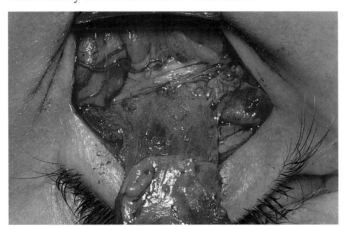

Fig. 9.4k

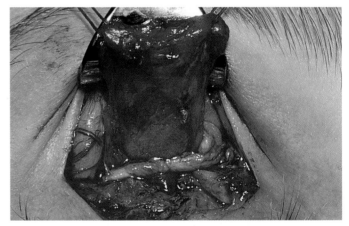

Fig. 9.4l

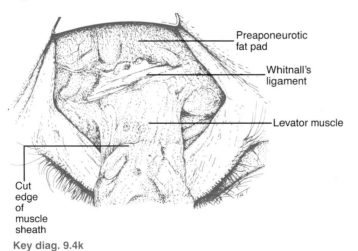

Preaponeurotic fat pad

Whitnall's ligament

Levator muscle

Cut edge of muscle sheath

Key diag. 9.4k

9:5　Posterior levator resection

9.5a

Expose the anterior surface of the levator aponeurosis and the septum as described in 9.3a–e.

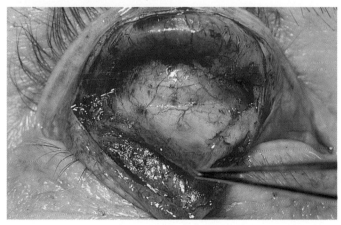

Fig. 9.5a

9.5b

Open the septum to expose the preaponeurotic fat pad and the anterior fibres of the levator muscle (arrow).

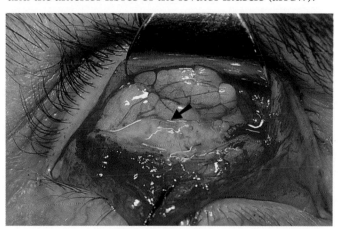

Fig. 9.5b

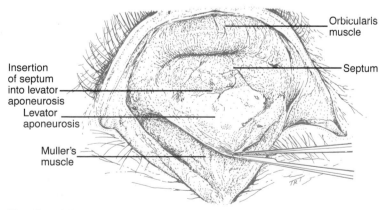

Orbicularis muscle

Septum

Insertion of septum into levator aponeurosis

Levator aponeurosis

Muller's muscle

Key diag. 9.5a

Technique continues overleaf →

9.5c

Retract the fat pad to confirm the position of Whitnall's ligament.

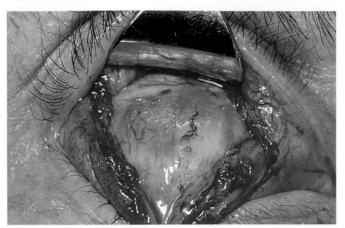

Fig. 9.5c

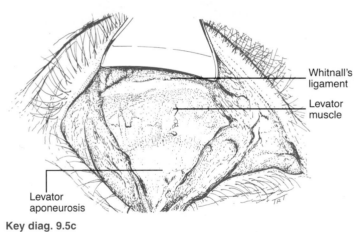

Key diag. 9.5c

Labels in diagram:
- Whitnall's ligament
- Levator muscle
- Levator aponeurosis

9.5d

With gentle downward traction on the cut conjunctival edge, dissect the levator and Muller's muscle from the conjunctiva as far as the superior fornix (see 9.4f). Identify the horns by transverse traction on the edge of the aponeurosis (see Fig. 9.4f) and cut them.

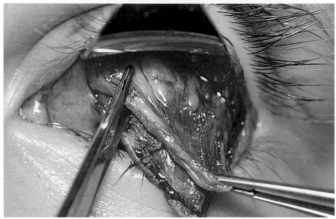

Fig. 9.5d

9.5e

Place double-armed 4/0 sutures as described in 9.3f–i.

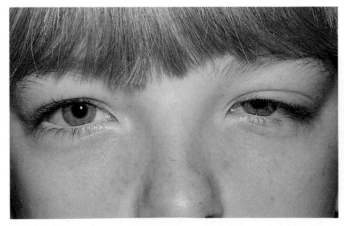

Fig. 9.5 pre

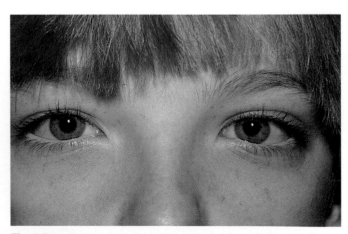

Fig. 9.5 post

Alternative procedure

Ptosis correction in oriental eyelids

The low skin crease in the Oriental upper lid is due to a low insertion of the levator aponeurosis into the orbicularis muscle close to the lash line (see 1.17). The orbital septum and the preaponeurotic fat pad also extend well inferiorly. The decision must be taken preoperatively about the desired skin crease level after operation. If it is to be raised and the lid 'westernised' make the incision at the intended level and excise the underlying septum and preaponeurotic fat overlying the tarsal plate. After the levator resection close the skin the usual way, taking deep bites into the anterior surface of the aponeurosis. If the skin crease is to remain low make the incision in the existing crease. The dissection to expose the levator aponeurosis is made deep to the septum with preservation of all the septum and the preaponeurotic fat. After resection of the levator close the skin directly.

If the posterior approach is preferred the sutures fixing the aponeurosis are brought through the tarsal plate in the usual way then inferiorly through the skin at the level of the low skin crease. If the lid is to be 'westernised' an anterior approach is preferable.

Complications and management

Overcorrection following a posterior approach is treated by removal of the sutures. If this is ineffective evert the lid over a Desmarres retractor and, if necessary, separate the wound edges at the superior border of the tarsal plate. Start downward traction on the lashes against forced upgaze three times daily and follow each treatment with 30 seconds of lid massage. Stop once the lids are level. If overcorrection persists, and especially if corneal exposure occurs, lower the lid surgically as described in Chapter 11.

Undercorrection may improve as oedema subsides. Wait 6 months and repeat the operation if the lid remains low.

A low skin crease may be improved by passing three double-armed 4/0 absorbable ('Pang') sutures from the conjunctiva just above the tarsus to the skin at the level of the new skin crease. They are removed after 3 weeks if they have not dissolved.

If the skin crease is high, or if there is a low crease in which Pang sutures have failed, make an incision at the level of the intended skin crease. Deepen it through the orbicularis muscle and free orbicularis from the tarsal plate and the levator aponeurosis for several millimetres either side of the incision. Create the new skin crease by closing the skin with sutures which pick up the deep layer – levator aponeurosis or tarsal plate – at the level of the crease.

Localised defects of the lid curve are treated by a tenotomy (for a peak) or a further small localised resection (for a flattening of the curve) over the area involved.

A lash ptosis results if the anterior lamellar tissues, below the skin crease, are too loose. Excessive eversion of the lashes or an ectropion of the upper lid may result from too tight an anterior lamella. To correct these reopen the skin crease and proceed as described for an abnormal skin crease. Reposition the anterior lamella correctly and resuture the wound with sutures which pick up the deep layer.

Prolapse of the conjunctiva is uncommon and most cases improve without treatment. Pang sutures may be needed if a prolapse persists.

Brow suspension

Choice of operation

Autogenous fascia lata (see 2.18) is the best material for a brow suspension. The ptosis may recur if a synthetic or homologous material is used. Fascia lata is difficult to remove from the small legs of very young children and an alternative is preferable in this age group, e.g. stored fascia lata, 2/0 monofilament nylon suture or Mersilene mesh. In these cases the Fox procedure (9.10) is chosen because any scarring will not interfere with later surgery if the ptosis recurs. In older children and adults the Crawford method (9.6) is preferred. A bilateral brow suspension is often recommended even though the ptosis is unilateral. If this is not done the difference in movement between the upper lids may be obviously asymmetrical postoperatively and less cosmetic. If, in addition, the levator function on the unaffected side is good it is advisable to weaken this levator (9.7) before inserting the suspension material. If this is not done the child may neglect to use the brow on the affected side, despite a bilateral brow suspension operation.

9:6   Fascia lata brow suspension – Crawford method

9.6a

Six short incisions about 3 mm long are made in the upper lid and brow on each side. The three lid incisions are placed immediately below the intended level of the skin crease. They should not be more than about 3 mm from the lid margin or their effectiveness in lifting the lid will be reduced. Mark the central one slightly nasal to the mid-point of the lid above the highest point of the lid margin. Mark the nasal one just lateral to the line of the punctum and the temporal one an equal distance to the lateral side of the central mark. Mark the medial and lateral brow incisions immediately above the brow and space them a little more widely apart than the equivalent lid incisions. Mark the final incision about 1–2 cm above the brow to create an isosceles triangle.

9.6b

Two strips of fascia are used on each side. Protect the eye. Using a Wright's fascia lata needle introduce the strips deep to the orbicularis muscle, on the surface of the tarsal plate.

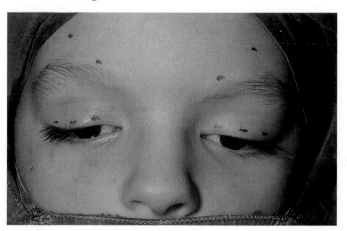

Fig. 9.6a

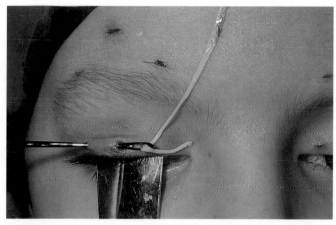

Fig. 9.6b

9.6c

Using the Wright's needle pull both ends of the lateral strip of fascia up to the lateral brow incision. Having introduced the Wright's needle into the brow incision pass it deep to orbicularis down to the lid incisions in turn.

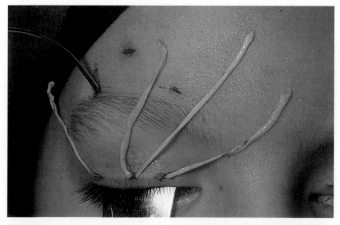

Fig. 9.6c

Technique continues overleaf →

9:6   **Fascia lata brow suspension – Crawford method** *(Continued)*

9.6d

Pull the ends of the other strip of fascia to the medial brow incision.

9.6e

Tie the strips at each brow incision to lift the lid. Reinforce the knots with a 6/0 absorbable suture. In general the lids should be lifted as high as possible in anticipation of a drop postoperatively. Stop if the lid level reaches the upper limbus or if an ectropion appears. (The exception to this rule is the occasional use of a brow suspension in ocular myopathies when the lids should be left closed on the table after the fascia is tied.)

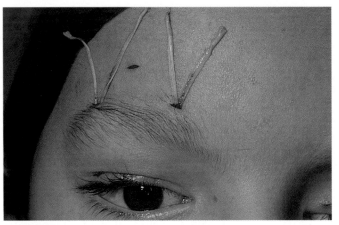

Fig. 9.6d

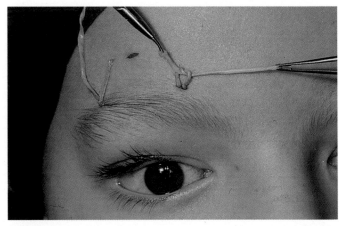

Fig. 9.6e

9.6f

Trim one of the two ends of fascia lata in each brow incision and pull the other up to the central forehead incision. The Wright's needle should be introduced down to the periosteum and then slightly withdrawn before passing it down to the brow incisions. In this way the fascial strips will be placed within the frontalis muscle. Tie the two ends of fascia at the forehead and reinforce the knot with a 6/0 absorbable suture. Before cutting this suture secure it to the subcutaneous tissues.

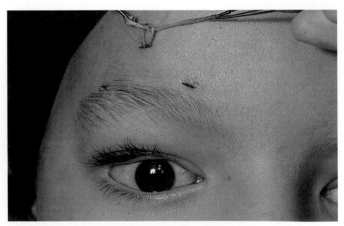

Fig. 9.6f

Fascia lata brow suspension – Crawford method

9.6g

Close the brow and forehead incisions with a 6/0 absorbable suture. No sutures are needed in the lid incisions which are buried in the skin creases. Insert Frost sutures.

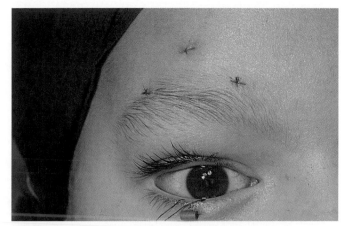

Fig. 9.6g

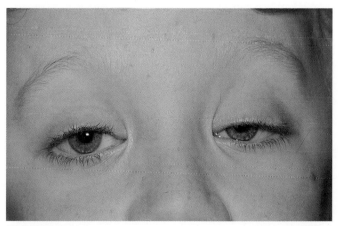

Fig. 9.6 pre A

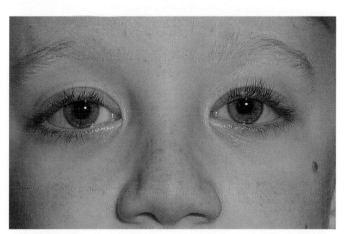

Fig. 9.6 post A

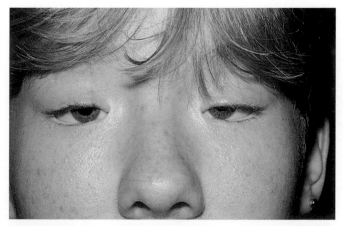

Fig. 9.6 pre B

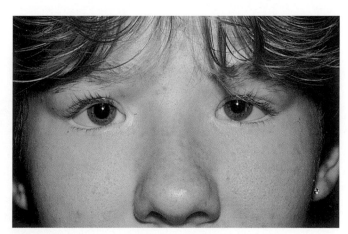

Fig. 9.6 post B

9:7   Levator weakening

See the comments in Section D ('Choice of operation').

9.7a

Expose the levator muscle and Whitnall's ligament from a posterior approach as described in 9.3a–e.

9.7b

With a Desmarres retractor in place identify, by gentle dissection, the borders of the levator muscle (arrow) above Whitnall's ligament. Carefully dissect immediately beneath the levator muscle to separate it from the underlying superior rectus muscle. Place a squint hook beneath the levator and perform a traction test on the globe to confirm that the superior rectus muscle has not been included.

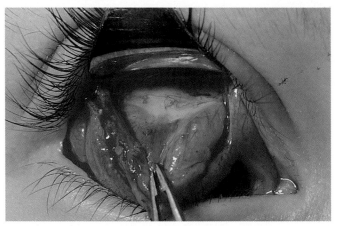

Fig. 9.7a

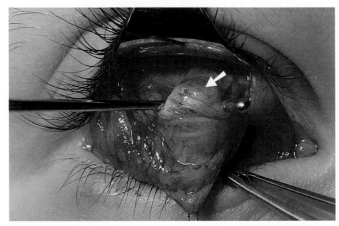

Fig. 9.7b

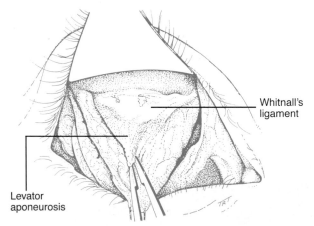

Whitnall's ligament

Levator aponeurosis

Key diag. 9.7a

9.7e

Close the conjunctiva with a continuous 6/0 absorbable suture.

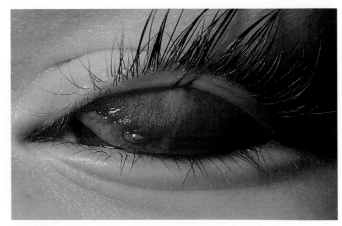

Fig. 9.7e

9.7c

Pass a second squint hook beneath the levator muscle to expose about 1cm of muscle.

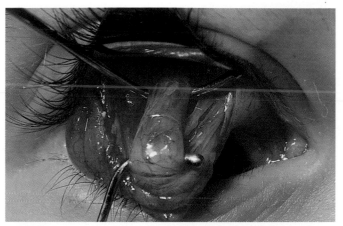

Fig. 9.7c

9.7d

Clamp the levator muscle with artery forceps proximal to the upper squint hook, remove the forceps and cauterise the muscle. Excise 1cm of muscle.

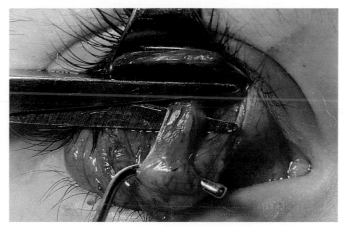

Fig. 9.7d

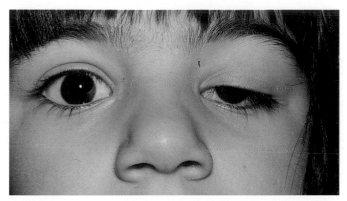

Fig. 9.7 pre

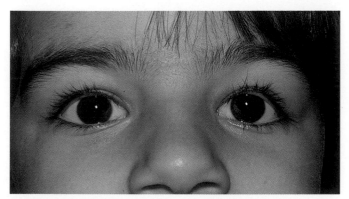

Fig. 9.7 post Right levator weakened. Bilateral brow suspension.

Complications and management

Marked overcorrection or undercorrection may be improved by adjustment to the fascia lata slings during the first 2 weeks postoperatively. If the asymmetry is mild wait for the swelling to subside and reassess. Once healing has occurred consider a repeat sling with autogenous fascia lata in 6 months if there is unacceptable asymmetry due to a low lid on one side. If the lid is high after healing has occurred make a skin crease incision and cut the slings. The lid may not drop significantly until the slings are dissected free from their surrounding tissues. Close the skin crease in the usual way (see 9.2h).

A poor lid curve or droop at one end of the lid are difficult to correct postoperatively and time should be taken during the operation to achieve the best curve. If the result is obviously not acceptable immediately postoperatively try to adjust the fascia lata slings. Later, allow full healing to occur and attempt to tuck the upper lid retractors and slings through a skin crease incision.

Alternative procedures

9:8 Anterior approach levator weakening

The levator may be excised through a skin approach as in anterior levator resection.

9:9 Levator transfer

Instead of excising the levator its action may be transferred to a fixed point so that it cannot act on the lid. Expose the anterior surface of the orbital septum as in an anterior levator resection, opening the septum. Dissect further superiorly along the anterior surface of the septum as far as the superior orbital rim. Open the septum to expose the levator muscle. Measure 15mm above the upper tarsal border, undermine the levator muscle and divide it. Dissect along the posterior surface of the levator to the upper fornix. Place three double-armed 6/0 non-absorbable sutures in the cut end of the levator and pass them through three small incisions in the septum close to the superior orbital rim. Pass the needles through the arcus marginalis and tie the sutures to fix the levator. Close the incisions in the septum to cover the cut end of the muscle. Close the skin crease incision in the usual way (see 9.2h).

Alte

9:11

An alter
procedu
the ante
drop ag

Expose
for an a

Insert th
Whitna
the tars
their po

9:10 Brow suspension – Fox method

Although this method of brow suspension may be used at any age we reserve its use for children who are too young to have fascia lata taken but who cannot wait to have the ptosis corrected because, for example, of amblyopia due to the ptotic lid. Stored fascia lata, a 2/0 monofilament suture or Mersilene mesh are possible substitutes for autogenous fascia lata.

9.10a

Mark two stab incisions in the lid 2 mm from the lash line and at the junctions of the inner and middle thirds, and middle and outer thirds, of the lid. Using a measuring caliper or forceps press on the marks to confirm that a satisfactory lid curve and skin crease are obtained. Adjust their position as necessary.

9.10b

Mark three stab incisions above the brow as for the Crawford technique (see 9.6a). Insert a corneal protector. Make stab incisions through all the marks using a sharp pointed blade such as a Bard Parker no. 11 blade. Using a Wright's fascia needle introduce a single length of the suspending material deep to the orbicularis muscle, first between the lid crease incisions.

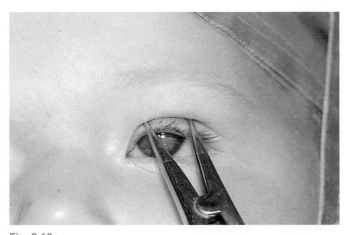

Fig. 9.10a

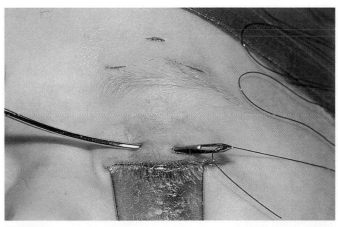

Fig. 9.10b

9.10c

Introduce the fascia lata needle through each brow incision in turn and draw the suspension material up to the brow.

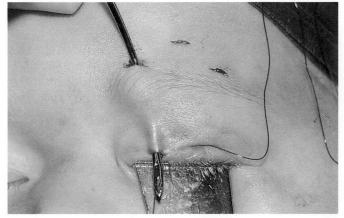

Fig. 9.10c   *Technique continues overleaf* ➔

FURTHER READING

Anderson R L, Jordan D R, Dutton J J: Whitnall's sling for poor function ptosis. Arch Ophthalmol 108: 1628; 1990

Callahan M, Beard C: Ptosis. Aesculapius Publishing Company, Birmingham, Alabama; 1990

Collin J R O: A ptosis repair of aponeurotic defects by the posterior approach. Br J Ophthalmol 63: 586; 1979

Crawford J S: Repair of ptosis using frontalis muscle and fascia lata: a 20 year review. Ophthalmol Surg 8: 31; 1977

Downes R N, Collin J R O: The mersilene mesh sling – a new concept in ptosis surgery. Br J Ophthalmol 73: 498; 1989

Fasanella R M, Servat J: Levator resection for minimal ptosis: another simplified operation: Arch Ophthalmol 65: 493; 1961

Frueh B R: The mechanistic classification of ptosis. Ophthalmology 87: 1019; 1980

Jones L T, Quickert M H, Wobig J L: The cure of ptosis by aponeurotic repair. Arch Ophthalmol 93: 629; 1975

CHAPTER 10

Blepharoplasty

Introduction

Blepharoplasty includes the removal of skin, muscle and fat in varying proportions from the eyelids. Widely different techniques have been described and the choice depends on the assessment of the individual patient and the preference of the surgeon. This chapter describes one approach to blepharoplasty and it should include enough basic information for other techniques to be evaluated.

Before removing an apparent excess of skin or fat from the upper or lower eyelids a careful preoperative assessment is essential with the patient sitting.

Preoperative assessment

Measure the visual acuity. Exclude the presence of a ptosis of either the upper lid or the brow. If there is a brow ptosis the brow must be held in its correct position for the remainder of the assessment (see 3.10). If there is blepharoptosis gently lift the excess upper lid skin to see whether the ptosis is corrected. If not, a true blepharoptosis exists. Note the position and degree of skin excess and fat prolapse. Measure the level of the skin crease (see 3.11). Assess laxity of the medial and lateral canthal tendons and overall laxity in the lower lid (see 3.12, 3.13). Examine the eye for disease of the cornea or conjunctiva. Assess the tear production (see 3.14a, b). Finally, discuss the patient's expectations so that the likely result of surgery is understood.

Choice of operation

If there is a brow ptosis this must be corrected (Sect. C) before the removal of any tissue from the upper lid. Blepharoptosis is corrected at the time of blepharoplasty (10.3).

The level and security of the upper lid skin crease is an important factor in the choice of blepharoplasty procedure in the upper lid (Sect. A).

Laxity of the lower lid must be corrected (see Ch. 7) either as a separate procedure or at the time of blepharoplasty if ectropion is to be avoided after lower lid blepharoplasty.

See also the Choice of operations under each section.

Classification:

Upper lid
– skin crease unsatisfactory ⎫ with or
– skin crease satisfactory ⎪ without
– blepharoptosis ⎬ fat
– brow ptosis ⎭ prolapse

Lower lid
– marked dermatochalasis ⎫ with or
– minimal dermatochalasis ⎪ without
– horizontal laxity ⎬ fat
– no horizontal laxity ⎭ prolapse

Upper lid blepharoplasty

The aim in upper lid blepharoplasty is to remove excess skin and muscle and prolapsed fat and to close the lid with a skin crease at a normal level of about 8–10 mm from the lashes in females, a little lower in men.

Choice of operation

Whether or not the skin crease is satisfactory, the surgical approach required to remove excess skin, muscle and fat is the same so these will be described first (10.1). The security and position of the skin crease determine the method of surgical closure of the lid (10.4). If the skin crease is already secure at a satisfactory level from the lash line it is not necessary to provide extra support for the skin crease by deep fixation to the tarsal plate or the levator aponeurosis above the tarsal plate. The skin may be closed edge to edge without deep fixation (10.4b). If, however, it is low, poorly secured (with anterior lamellar slippage downwards) or is unsatisfactory in any way a new skin crease is created at the correct level and supported by deep fixation sutures (10.4a). These usually also close the skin but some surgeons prefer to place them deeply before skin closure. If a ptosis is present this is corrected at the same operation (10.3).

Dressings after blepharoplasty

Eye pads may be applied for about an hour. They may then be removed and ice packs applied gently to the closed eyelids to reduce tissue swelling. If there is pain the pads must be removed immediately to exclude a compressive orbital haemorrhage.

10:1 **Skin and muscle excision**

10.1a

Mark the existing skin crease, if satisfactory, or a new one 7–10 mm from the lash line, if unsatisfactory. Extend the mark from a point above the punctum to the lateral canthus and extend the mark laterally and upwards at about 45 degrees as far as the orbital rim.

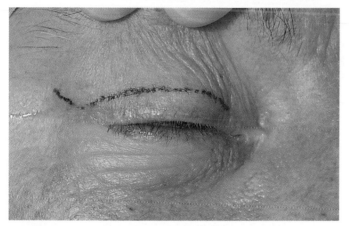

Fig. 10.1a

10.1b

Ask the patient to look down with both eyes open. Using forceps based at the skin crease gently estimate the excess skin at a number of sites. Aim to remove just enough skin to leave the lid closed or, at most, to result in slight eversion of the lid margin.

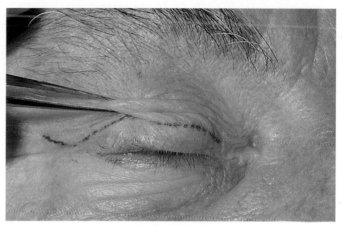

Fig. 10.1b

10.1c

At each site mark the upper limit of the skin to be excised and join the marks. Extend this line downwards medially and upwards laterally to join the first line at each end.

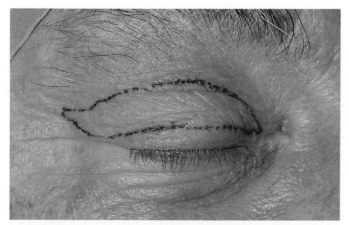

Fig. 10.1c

10.1d

Excise the marked area of skin, being careful to leave the orbicularis muscle intact.

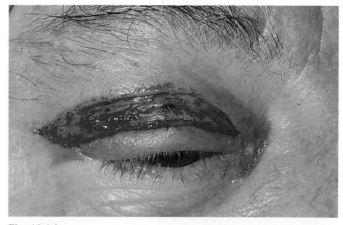

Fig. 10.1d

Technique continues overleaf →

Excise a strip of orbicularis muscle, 5–6 mm wide, from just above the lower wound edge. Excise more muscle if there is a marked excess.

10.1f

Excision of the strip of orbicularis muscle exposes the superior border of the tarsal plate, the lower part of the levator aponeurosis and the lower part of the orbital septum. Press gently on the closed eye or lower lid to accentuate any prolapse of fat from the medial and central fat compartments. Excise excess fat (10.2) and correct any ptosis (10.3), then decide on the type of skin closure (10.4).

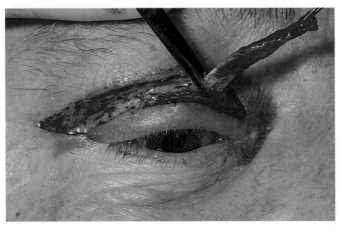

Fig. 10.1e

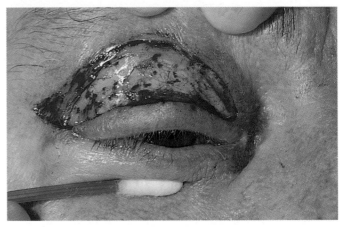

Fig. 10.1f

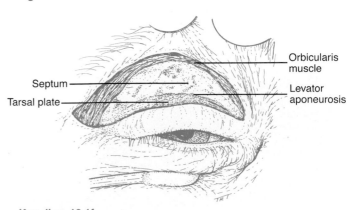

Key diag. 10.1f

10:2   Fat excision or cautery

Either excise the excess fat or apply cautery to it through the septum. If a ptosis is to be corrected the septum is opened fully and fat excision is then preferred.

10.2a

To excise the fat through an unopened septum make small incisions in the septum with sharp pointed scissors and allow the fat of the central and medial compartments to prolapse.

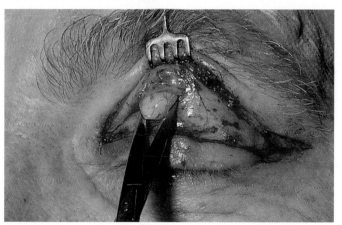

Fig. 10.2a

10.2b

Apply fine curved artery forceps and excise redundant fat without traction. Cauterise the cut edge then remove the forceps and apply more cautery before allowing the fat to fall back into the orbit.

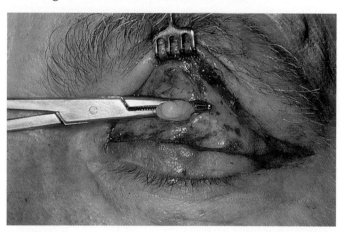

Fig. 10.2b

10.2c

If cautery is preferred it should be applied in several rows across the unopened septum. A bipolar diathermy or a hand-held battery cautery is preferred, to avoid any risk of damage to posterior orbital structures.

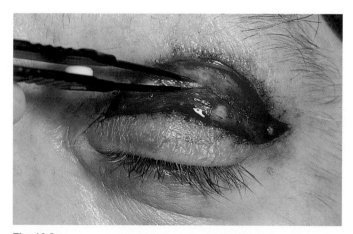

If a ptosis is present it should now be corrected (10.3). If there is no ptosis the skin is now closed (10.4).

Fig. 10.2c

10:3 Ptosis correction

The ptosis associated with an eyelid requiring a blepharoplasty will almost always be of the aponeurotic disinsertion type.

10.3a

Having exposed the septum (see 10.1a–f) open it transversely (see 9.2c, d).

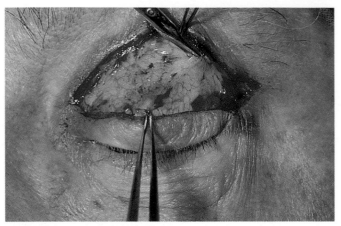

Fig. 10.3a

10.3b

The preaponeurotic fat pad is exposed. The medial fat pad lies medially. Excise excess fat from the central and medial fat pads (see 10.2b).

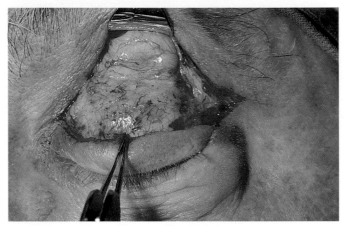

Fig. 10.3b

10.3d

With a minimum of dissection advance the healthy aponeurosis to the tarsal plate and secure it with a temporary suture. Check the lid level by asking the patient to look up and down. If it is low some aponeurosis may need to be resected. Place two further sutures (arrow) in the aponeurosis to achieve a satisfactory lid margin contour.

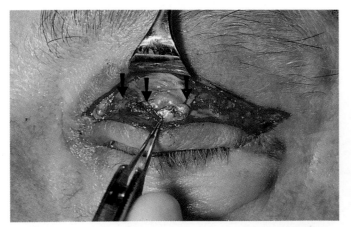

Fig. 10.3d

10.3e

Close the lid with deep fixation as described in 10.4a.

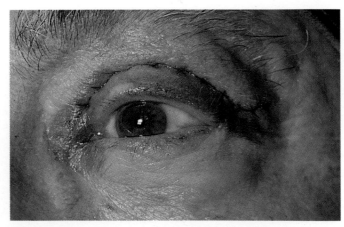

Fig. 10.3e

10.3c

Identify healthy aponeurotic tissue.

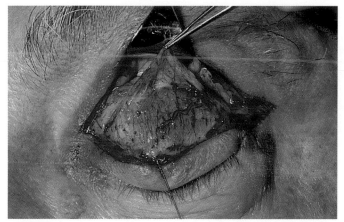

Fig. 10.3c

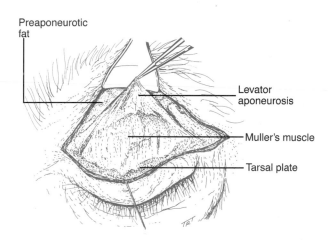

Preaponeurotic fat

Levator aponeurosis

Muller's muscle

Tarsal plate

Key diag. 10.3c

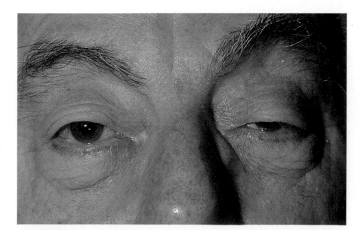

Fig. 10.3 pre

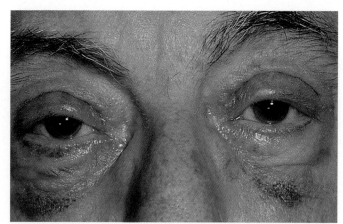

Fig. 10.3 post

10:4 | Skin closure

10.4a | With deep fixation

This technique is used if the skin crease is less than 7–9 mm from the lashes or if it is absent, double, poorly fixed or unsatisfactory in any way and a new skin crease must be created (see Figs 10.3 Pre/Post).

Having completed the excision of skin, muscle and fat (10.1 and 10.2) and corrected any ptosis (10.3), close the skin, with deep attachment to the levator aponeurosis, with interrupted 6/0 sutures (see 9.2h). Remove the sutures at 5 days.

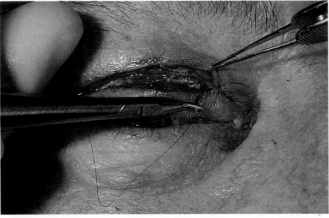

Fig. 10.4a A

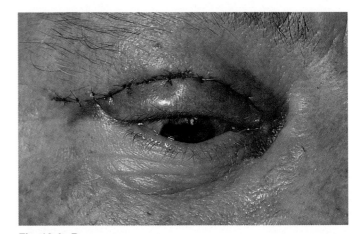

Fig. 10.4a B

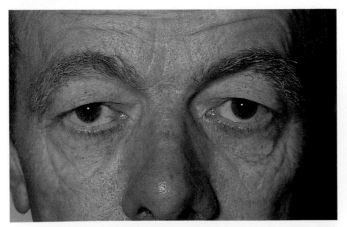

Fig. 10.4 pre

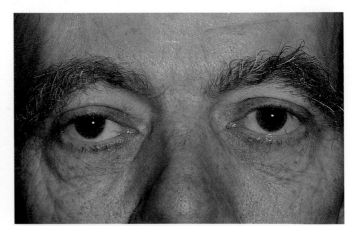

Fig. 10.4 post

10.4b Without deep fixation

This technique is used if the skin crease is secure at a satisfactory level from the lash line.

Close the skin edge to edge without deep attachment to the levator aponeurosis or tarsal plate. Use a continuous 6/0 non-absorbable suture, which may be subcuticular, for the lid crease and interrupted sutures in the oblique part of the wound laterally.

10.4c

If there is excess skin remaining medially make an oblique incision upwards and medially from the medial end of the wound, undermine and excise the excess.

Complications and management

The most serious, although uncommon, early complication of upper lid blepharoplasty is haemorrhage following excision of orbital fat. If persistent the pressure of the resulting haematoma may threaten vision. Blindness, however, is very rare. This complication can be prevented by avoiding traction on the orbital fat during fat excision and careful attention to haemostasis. A serious haematoma occurring during the hours following surgery should be evacuated by reopening the lid.

Oedema of the lid tissues is common and may be reduced by ice packs during the hours following surgery.

Discomfort in the eyes from exposure is not uncommon in the first weeks after blepharoplasty but it should settle with no more than topical lubricants. More serious complications of exposure, such as corneal ulcers, are rare.

Milia occasionally form along the skin crease. They may be removed individually if they do not disappear within a few months.

Webbing may occur between the upper and lower lid scars if they are closer laterally than 4mm. A Z-plasty may be needed to correct the web.

Altered pigmentation may occur in the scars. In time this usually improves.

Following blepharoplasty the dressings should be removed about an hour after surgery and ice packs applied to the closed lids for 2–3 hours to reduce oedema. Remove all sutures at 5 days.

Lower lid blepharoplasty

The aim in lower lid blepharoplasty is to excise any excess skin, muscle and fat, being careful to avoid a postoperative ectropion. This complication may occur if too much skin is excised or if there is horizontal lower lid laxity. The cause of horizontal laxity may be medial or lateral canthal tendon laxity or generalised lid laxity (see 3.12, 3.13).

Choice of operation

Canthal tendon laxity must be corrected first (see 7.4, 7.5). Generalised laxity without significant laxity in the canthal tendons is corrected as part of the blepharoplasty (see below). In the older patient with thin lower lid skin and poor tone in the orbicularis muscle choose a skin flap blepharoplasty (10.5). In a younger patient, especially if there is fat prolapse but minimal excess skin, a skin-muscle flap blepharoplasty is preferred (10.6).

10:5 Skin flap blepharoplasty

This technique is used in the older patient with thin lower lid skin and poor lid muscle tone. It is very similar to the Kuhnt–Zymanowski procedure for ectropion (see 7.3).

10.5a

Mark the incision 1–2mm below the lashes from the punctum to the lateral canthus. Extend the line laterally and slightly downwards in a laugh line as far as the orbital rim. This line should be at least 4mm from the lateral end of an upper lid blepharoplasty incision.

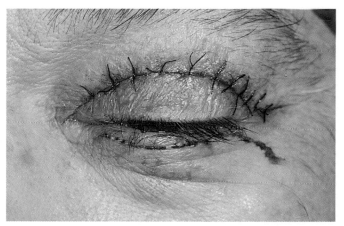

Fig. 10.5a

10.5b

Dissect the skin flap from the underlying orbicularis muscle as far as the inferior orbital rim. If there is horizontal lid laxity tighten the lid by excision of a full thickness pentagon centrally (see 2.6). If there is an obvious excess of orbicularis muscle excise a narrow strip just inferior to the tarsal plate. Before repairing the defect in the muscle with loosely tied 6/0 absorbable sutures, press gently on the closed eye to accentuate any fat herniation.

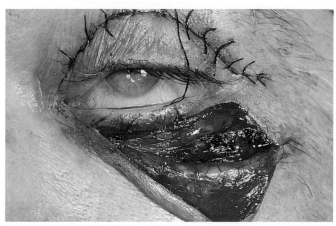

Fig. 10.5b

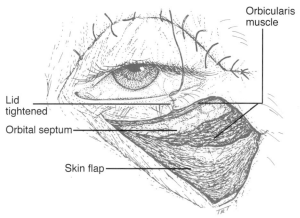

Orbicularis muscle

Lid tightened

Orbital septum

Skin flap

Key diag. 10.5b

Technique continues overleaf ➔

10:5   **Skin flap blepharoplasty** *(Continued)*

10.5c

Excess fat is now removed from the central, medial and lateral fat pads as necessary. If a strip of orbicularis muscle has been excised the septum has been exposed and the fat may be cauterised through the closed septum.

Alternatively, excise excess fat as in the upper lid (see 10.2a,b). Repair the defect in the orbicularis with absorbable 6/0 sutures. If the orbicularis is intact make short horizontal incisions through the muscle just above the inferior orbital rim by spreading scissors over the sites of fat herniation. Note that the lateral fat pad is placed slightly superior as well as lateral to the central fat pad. Excise the fat, without traction, as described in 10.2b above (see also 10.6c, d).

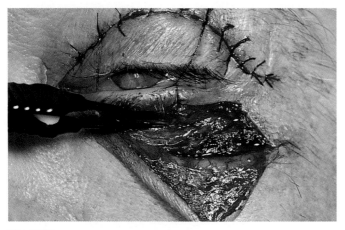

Fig. 10.5c

10.5f

Close the skin with a continuous 6/0 monofilament suture along the lid and interrupted sutures lateral to the canthus. Remove the sutures in 5 days.

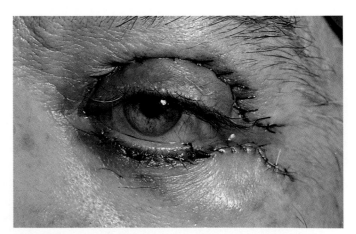

Fig. 10.5f

10.5d

Ask the patient to look up and open the mouth. Drape the skin flap over the lid margin with gentle upward and lateral traction. Excise any excess by first making a horizontal incision to remove the vertical excess.

10.5e

Then excise the lateral triangle of excess skin.

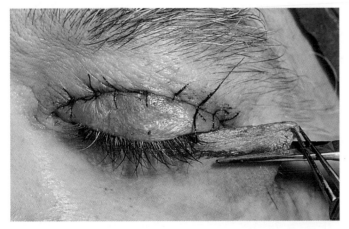

Fig. 10.5d

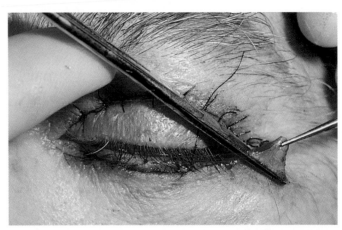

Fig. 10.5e

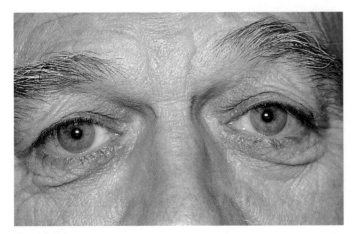

Fig. 10.5 pre

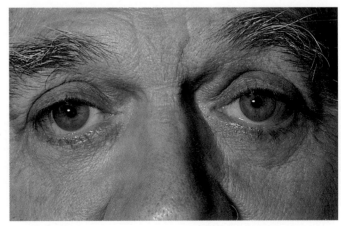

Fig. 10.5 post

10:6   Skin-muscle flap blepharoplasty

This technique is used in the younger patient, especially if there is fat herniation but minimal excess skin.

10.6a	**10.6b**
Mark the incision as described in 10.5a above.	Deepen the incision through the orbicularis muscle to the tarsal plate and extend it laterally as marked. Dissect the orbicularis muscle from the underlying orbital septum as far as the inferior orbital rim. Tighten the lid, if indicated.

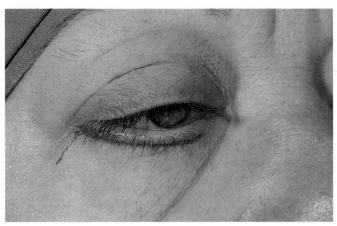

Fig. 10.6a

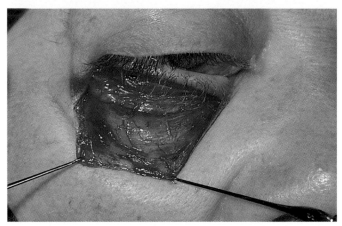

Fig. 10.6b

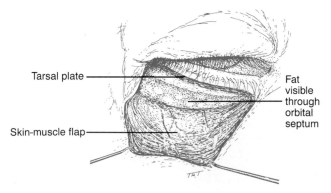

Tarsal plate

Fat visible through orbital septum

Skin-muscle flap

Key diag. 10.6b

10.6c

Press gently on the closed eye to accentuate fat herniation and make incisions in the septum over the sites of maximum herniation (see 10.2a).

10.6d

Excise excess fat, without traction (see 10.2b).

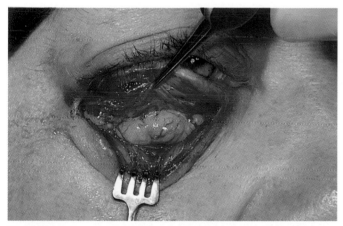

Fig. 10.6c

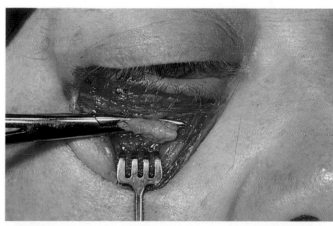

Fig. 10.6d

10.6e

There is usually relatively little excess skin to excise. Ask the patient to look up and open the mouth. Drape the skin-muscle flap over the lid margin with gentle upward and lateral traction. Excise excess, if any, by first making a horizontal incision to remove the vertical excess.

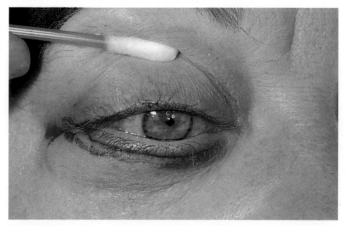

Fig. 10.6e

Technique continues overleaf →

10:6 **Skin-muscle flap blepharoplasty** (Continued)

10.6f

Then excise the triangle of excess skin and muscle laterally. Take care not to remove too much.

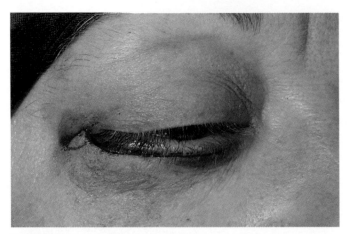

Fig. 10.6f

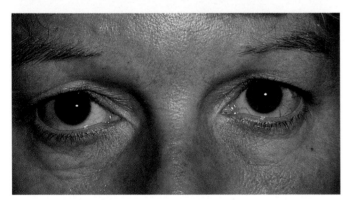

Fig. 10.6 pre

10.6g

Close the skin with a continuous 6/0 monofilament suture along the lid and interrupted sutures laterally. Remove all sutures at 5 days.

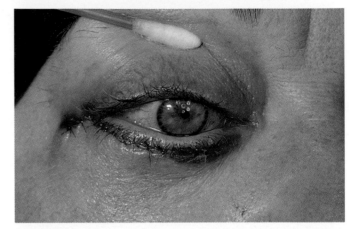

Fig. 10.6g

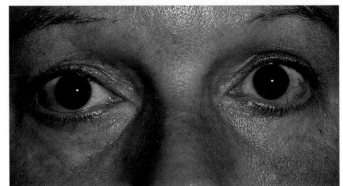

Fig. 10.6 post

Complications and management

In addition to the complications discussed above the main complication following lower lid blepharoplasty is ectropion. This occurs if too much skin is removed or if there is uncorrected horizontal lid laxity. It is prevented by tightening a lax lid at the time of the blepharoplasty and postoperative laxity is treated in the same way. However, if too much skin has been removed it may be necessary to insert a full thickness skin graft.

Brow ptosis

An eyebrow may droop as a result of involutional change or following a lower motor neurone facial nerve palsy. If there is reasonable function in the frontalis muscle, shortening the muscle and removing lax skin elevates the eyebrow effectively. If, however, the function in the frontalis muscle is poor, the brow must be anchored to the periosteum.

10:7 Whole brow elevation

10.7a

With the brow in its ptotic position mark the full length of its upper border. Pull the brow up to its intended position and hold the marker pen above the forehead skin at this level.

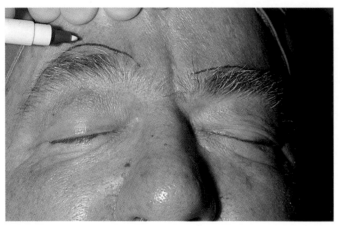

Fig. 10.7a

10.7b

With the marker pen held at the intended brow level allow the brow to drop again then mark the forehead skin. Repeat this manoeuvre at several sites along the brow to estimate the amount of skin, subcutaneous tissue and muscle to be resected.

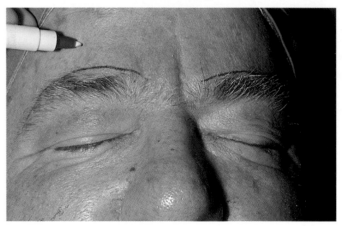

Fig. 10.7b

10.7d

Incise along the mark taking care to cut at right angles to the skin. Deepen the incision through the subcutaneous tissue and the thin frontalis muscle/epicranial aponeurosis layer until the loose underlying areolar connective tissue is reached superficial to the periosteum. Bleeding is often brisk. Take care to identify the supraorbital nerve and vessels as they pass superiorly from the supraorbital notch. Excise the skin ellipse, dissecting in the loose areolar tissue layer.

Close the wound in three layers. If the muscle is functioning the deepest layer is placed between the cut edges of the frontalis muscle/epicranial aponeurosis layer, just superficial to the loose areolar tissue. If the muscle is paralysed the deepest layer of sutures is between the deepest layer of the eyebrow tissues inferiorly and the periosteum at the level of the upper wound edge superiorly. In either case insert several non-absorbable 4/0 sutures.

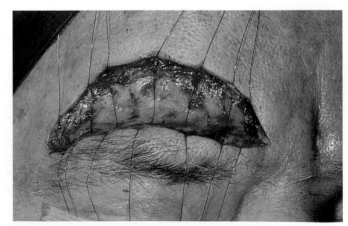

Fig. 10.7d

10.7c

Join the marks to form an ellipse.

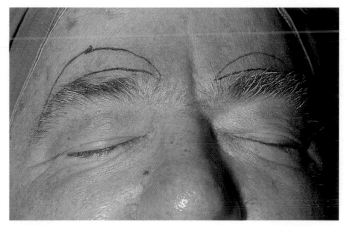

Fig. 10.7c

10.7e

Close the subcutaneous layer with 4/0 or 6/0 chromic catgut sutures. It is important to leave no 'dead space' deep to the final skin closure or an obvious sunken scar will result.

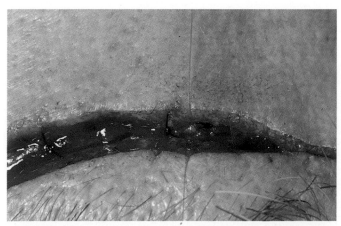

Fig. 10.7e

Technique continues overleaf →

10:7 **Whole brow elevation** *(Continued)*

10.7f

Close the skin with interrupted sutures of 4/0 silk or
nylon or a continuous subcuticular nylon. If
interrupted sutures are used they must be removed in
3–4 days to avoid suture marks. Remove a subcuticular
suture at 5 days.

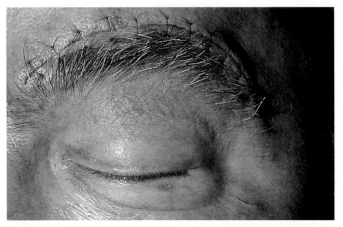

Fig. 10.7f

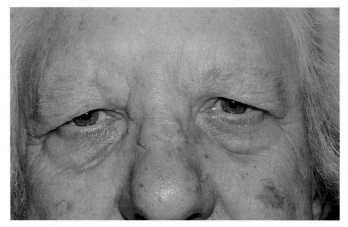

Fig. 10.7 pre

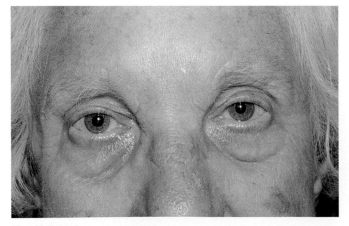

Fig. 10.7 post

Complications and management

Undercorrection is common as the brows tend to
drop again. The scars may be rather obvious if
care is not taken with closure. The most serious
complication is damage to the supraorbital nerve
resulting in numbness or paraesthesiae in the
forehead. This may be permanent. It can be
prevented if the nerve is identified and avoided,
especially with the cautery.

10:8 Lateral brow elevation

Ptosis of the lateral end of the brow may occur without
general brow ptosis. This can be corrected effectively
by removing an ellipse of skin and muscle based on a
lateral forehead skin crease.

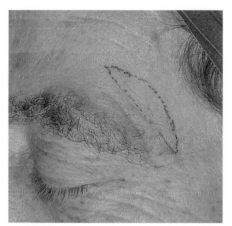

Fig. 10.8

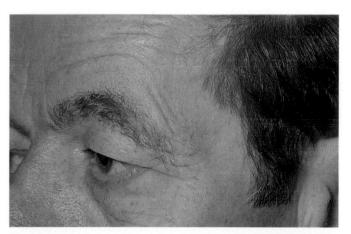

Fig. 10.8 pre

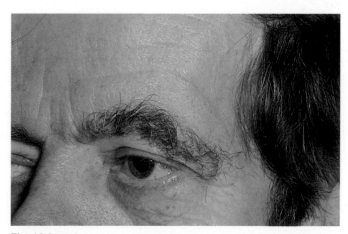

Fig. 10.8 post

FURTHER READING

Baylis H I, Long J A, Groth M J: Transconjunctival lower eyelid blepharoplasty. Ophthalmology 96: 1027; 1989

Bosniak S L, Sachs M E: Lipolytic diathermy. Orbit 4: 157, 1988

Bosniak S L: Cosmetic blepharoplasty. Raven Press, New York 1990

Chen W P: Asian blepharoplasty. Update on anatomy and techniques. Opthalm Plast Reconstr Surg 3: 135; 1987

Goldberg R A, Marmor M F et al: Blindness following blepharoplasty: two case reports and a discussion on management. Ophthalmic Surg 21: 85; 1990

Leone C R: Management of the blepharoplasty patient with ptosis. Ophthalmic Surg 19: 515; 1988

McCord C D, Doxanas M T: Browplasty and browpexy: an adjunct to blepharoplasty. Plast Reconstr Surg 86: 248; 1990

Parkes M, Fein W, Brennan H G: Pinch technique for repair of cosmetic eyelid deformities. Arch Ophthalmol 89: 324; 1973

Putterman A M: Cosmetic oculoplastic surgery. Grune and Stratton, New York; 1982

Sheen J H: Supratarsal fixation in upper blepharoplasty. Plast Reconstr Surg 54: 424; 1974

Shorr N, Seiff S R: Cosmetic blepharoplasty. An illustrated surgical guide. Slack Inc, Thorofare, New Jersey; 1986

CHAPTER 11

Eyelid retraction

Introduction

Corneal exposure is the most serious sequel to eyelid retraction. It may also occur with the eyelids in a normal position if there is poor closure or reduced tear production. In these situations, or if there is cosmetic asymmetry, even without exposure, an upper lid may need to be lowered or a lower lid raised.

Classification: Retraction with – no shortage of skin or conjunctiva
– shortage of skin
– shortage of conjunctiva

Choice of operation

If the lid retraction is due only to a shortage of skin an ectropion as well as retraction of the lid is likely. The treatment is a skin graft or a Z-plasty (see Ch. 7).

If the retraction is due to cicatricial changes in the conjunctiva an entropion also results and lengthening of the posterior lamella is necessary (see Ch. 6).

The procedures described in this chapter are appropriate if there is no shortage of the skin or the conjunctiva – the retraction is due to shortened lid retractors.

In the upper lid excise Muller's muscle alone to achieve a lid drop of about 2 mm (11.1). Recess both Muller's muscle and the levator aponeurosis to achieve about 3 mm (11.2, 11.3). The use of a spacer in either the upper lid (11.4, 11.5) or the lower lid (11.7) allows 4 mm or more of correction. An alternative to retractor recession is myotomy (11.6).

Muller's muscle

11:1 Muller's muscle excision

11.1a

Insert a traction suture, into the upper lid and evert the lid over a Desmarres retractor. Make a short, full thickness incision close to the upper border of the tarsal plate (arrows).

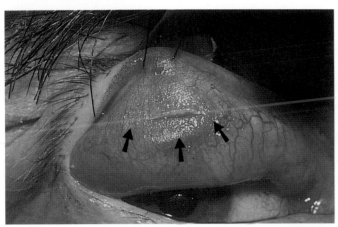

Fig. 11.1a

11.1b

Extend the incision medially and laterally, keeping parallel to the lid margin, to the full width of the tarsus.

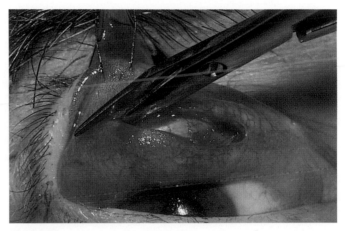

Fig. 11.1b

11.1c

Reflect the thin strip of superior tarsal border down towards the eye and identify Muller's muscle – a thin, rather vascular sheet of muscle inserting into the strip of tarsus. Dissect upwards in the fine connective tissue between Muller's muscle posteriorly and the levator aponeurosis anteriorly for about 10–12 mm until the origin of Muller's muscle from the levator is reached (see also 9.3 a–c).

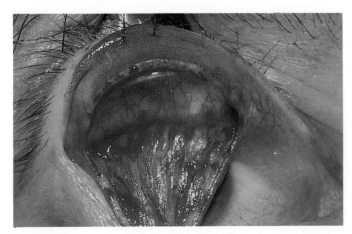

Fig. 11.1c

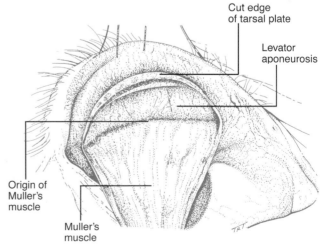

Key diag. 11.1c

Cut edge
of tarsal plate

Levator
aponeurosis

Origin of
Muller's
muscle

Muller's
muscle

Technique continues overleaf →

11:1 **Muller's muscle excision** *(Continued)*

11.1d

Now dissect the insertion of Muller's muscle free from the strip of tarsus, and from the underlying conjunctiva, as far as its origin.

11.1e

Divide Muller's muscle at this level and remove it taking care that no muscle fibres remain between the origin and the insertion.

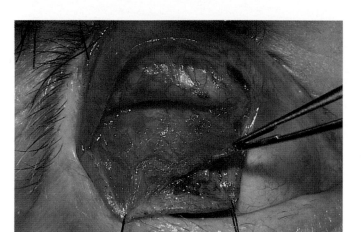

Fig. 11.1d

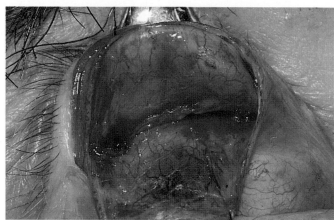

Fig. 11.1e

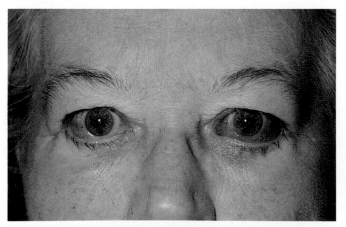

Fig. 11.1 pre

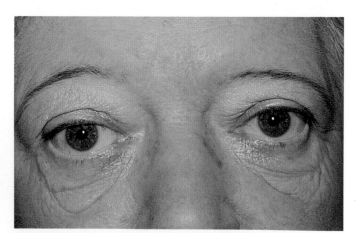

Fig. 11.1 post

11.1f

Excise the strip of tarsus and close the conjunctiva to the cut border of the tarsal plate with a continuous 6/0 absorbable suture. The knots should be buried. Tape a traction suture to the cheek for 48 hours (see 2.19b).

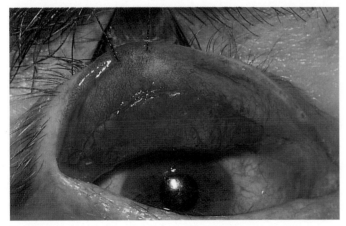

Fig. 11.1f

Complications and management

If Muller's muscle has been incompletely excised retraction in part of the lid will persist resulting in a poor curve. If marked, the remaining fibres should be excised.

Recession of Muller's muscle and levator

Choice of operation

If a spacer is not used a posterior approach (11.2) is easier but the skin crease will be raised in relation to the lashes. This is not important in bilateral cases but the resulting asymmetry in unilateral cases may be uncosmetic. To avoid this use an anterior approach to recess the upper lid retractors (11.3) and set the skin crease at the level of the opposite side. If the anterior approach is used excess fat and/or skin may be easily excised.

If a spacer is used the anterior approach to the levator (11.4) is usually preferred but the posterior approach (11.5) may be used.

11:2 Upper lid retractor recession without spacer – posterior approach

11.2a

Evert the upper lid and incise the tarsal plate as described in 11.1a, b above.

11.2b

Deepen the incision through the levator aponeurosis to expose the orbicularis muscle (see 9.3b–d). Dissect superiorly between the levator aponeurosis and the orbicularis muscle (see 9.3e), a few millimetres at a time, reassessing the lid position at each step. Aim at a slight overcorrection.

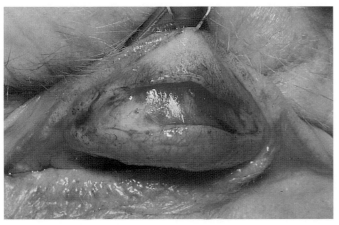

Fig. 11.2a

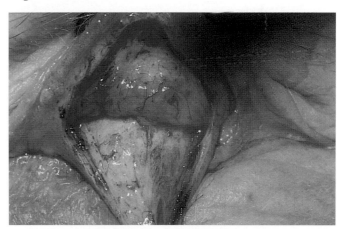

Fig. 11.2b

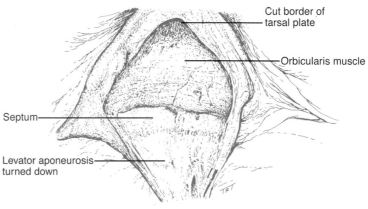

Key diag. 11.2b

In thyroid lid retraction the lateral end of the lid may remain high. See the comment in 11.3d.

Technique continues overleaf →

11:2 **Upper lid retractor recession without spacer – posterior approach** *(Continued)*

11.2c

The upper lid retractors and the conjunctiva may be sutured (although this is not essential) to the orbicularis muscle in their recessed position using continuous or interrupted 6/0 plain catgut. Try to bury the knots. Insert a traction suture (see 2.19b, 11.3d) and tape it to the cheek for 48 hours.

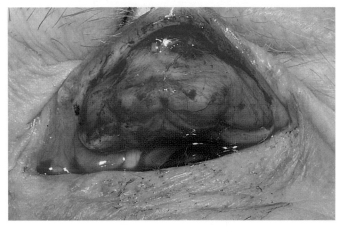

Fig. 11.2c

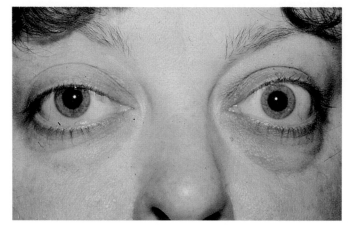

Fig. 11.2 pre

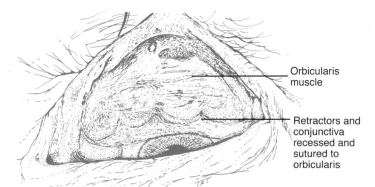

Orbicularis muscle

Retractors and conjunctiva recessed and sutured to orbicularis

Key diag. 11.2c

Upper lid retractor recession without spacer – posterior approach

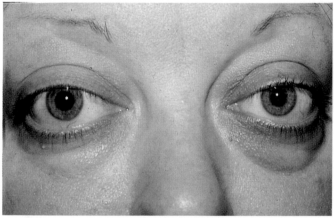

Fig. 11.2 post

Complications and management

If the retraction is undercorrected lid massage and traction on the lashes with upgaze may lower the lid further during the first 4–6 postoperative weeks. Reoperation will be needed if this is ineffective. If the lid is too low wait for 6 weeks to see how much it will rise. If it stays too low advance the retractors and resuture to the orbicularis muscle at the correct position.

A poor lid curve which does not resolve will require local adjustment to the position of part of the retractors.

11:3   Upper lid retractor recession without spacer – anterior approach

11.3a

Place a traction suture in the upper lid and make a skin crease incision. Expose the levator aponeurosis and orbital septum (see 9.2a–c).

11.3b

Dissect out the upper lid retractors (see 9.4e, f) so that they can retract allowing the tarsal plate to move downwards.

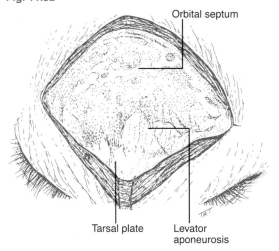

Fig. 11.3a

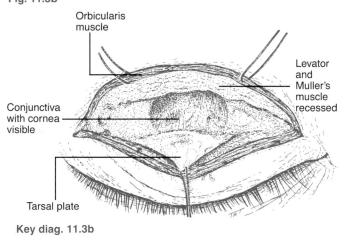

Fig. 11.3b

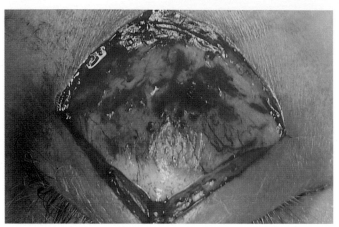

Key diag. 11.3a

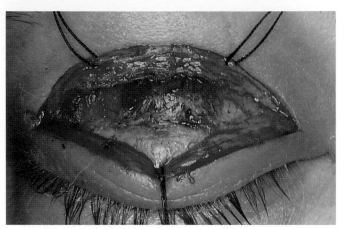

Key diag. 11.3b

Note – If the level of the skin crease is to be changed it is important to dissect free the insertion of the levator aponeurosis into the orbicularis muscle (at the level of the original skin crease) to avoid a double skin crease. Having done this open the septum and allow the preaponeurotic fat pad to prolapse to the level of the new skin crease to discourage reattachment.

A marked excess of fat in the medial and central compartments may be excised if necessary (see 10.2).

Upper lid retractor recession without spacer – anterior approach

11.3c

Assess the lid level by asking the patient to look up and down. Aim at a small overcorrection. Continue to dissect anterior and posterior to the retractors until a satisfactory level is achieved.

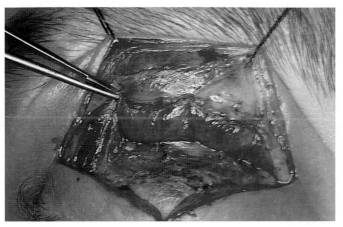

Fig. 11.3c

11.3d

Close the lid taking deep bites into the tarsal plate (see 9.2h). Insert a traction suture (see 2.19b) and tape it to the cheek for 48 hours.

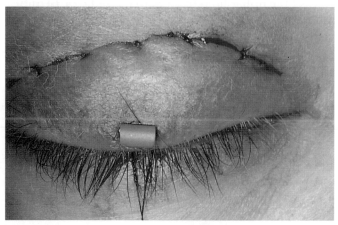

Fig. 11.3d

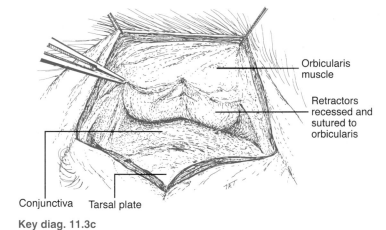

Orbicularis muscle

Retractors recessed and sutured to orbicularis

Conjunctiva   Tarsal plate

Key diag. 11.3c

Note – In retraction due to thyroid eye disease the lateral end of the lid is often difficult to lower to a satisfactory level. In these cases cut the lateral horn of the levator and reassess. If the lid is still high laterally cut the lateral end of Whitnall's ligament and continue to free the tissues laterally, taking care to avoid damage to the lacrimal gland, until a satisfactory curve is achieved.

The levator aponeurosis and Muller's muscle may be sutured (although this is not essential) to the orbicularis muscle, in their recessed position, with continuous or interrupted 6/0 plain catgut.

Complications and management

As for the posterior approach above. In addition, despite every effort, the lateral end of the lid may still be high. Wait 6 months and attempt to divide the lateral tissue further if necessary. If a double skin crease results despite the precautions described above (11.3b) it may be possible to eliminate it by further dissection between the orbicularis muscle and the levator at the level of the original (higher) crease.

Alternative procedures

11:5 Upper lid retractor recession with spacer – posterior approach

With the upper lid everted make an incision close to the upper border of the tarsal plate, incise the levator aponeurosis and dissect the anterior surface of the levator free, opening the septum, as described for a posterior levator resection (see 9.3). Cut the lateral horn of the aponeurosis (see 9.5d) and, if necessary, the lateral end of Whitnall's ligament. Dissect the conjunctiva free from Muller's muscle as far as the fornix. Allow the retractors to recess until a satisfactory lid level is achieved. Prepare a spacer as described in 11.4b above and suture its superior border to the recessed retractors using continuous 6/0 plain catgut. Suture the conjunctiva, together with the inferior border of the spacer, to the upper border of the tarsal plate using continuous 6/0 plain catgut. Insert a traction suture and tape it to the cheek for 48 hours.

Complications and management

As for 11.2 and 11.4

11:6 Levator Z-myotomy

Make an incision at the intended level of the skin crease and expose the anterior surface of the upper lid retractors (see 9.2a–c). Identify Whitnall's ligament and cut it at either side of the levator. Carefully dissect in the connective tissue either side of the levator to expose the medial and lateral borders of the muscle and the horns. Separate Muller's muscle from the conjunctiva by spreading with scissors. (If difficulty is encountered from the anterior side this may be done through a small incision in the conjunctiva close to the upper tarsal border, having injected local anaesthetic to separate the layers.) Pass a muscle hook beneath the belly of the levator proximal to Whitnall's ligament taking care to avoid damage to the underlying superior rectus muscle. Make a lateral transverse cut in the levator muscle, proximal to Whitnall's ligament, which extends for more than half its width. Make a similar cut from the medial side of the muscle (or aponeurosis) about 1 cm inferior to the first cut and distal to Whitnall's ligament. This lower cut must include Muller's muscle. The lid should be lowered by twice the amount of retraction and the length of the two cuts may be increased until this is achieved. If the lateral end of the lid remains inadequately corrected make a third cut from the lateral border of the aponeurosis and Muller's muscle.

Allow the preaponeurotic fat to prolapse to the level of the skin crease and close the skin incision with interrupted 6/0 sutures which pass through the anterior surface of the levator aponeurosis. Insert a traction suture and tape it to the cheek for 48 hours.

Complications and management

The lid will be swollen and ptotic postoperatively. During the first six weeks it will rise to its final level. If the level remains too low wait 6 months and adjust the level, if necessary, as described for the correction of ptosis by the anterior approach (see 9.4). If it is too high an alternative method of lid lowering should be used after 6 months to achieve the desired level.

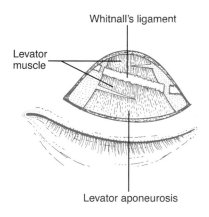

Whitnall's ligament

Levator muscle

Levator aponeurosis

Diag. 11.1a

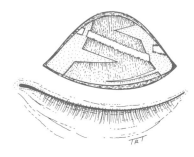

Diag. 11.1b

Lower lid

11:7 Recession of lower lid retractors

The conjunctival approach is easiest for the lower lid and a spacer, although not essential, gives a more predictable result.

11.7a

Insert one or two traction sutures and evert the lid over a Desmarres retractor. Make an incision in the conjunctiva just inferior to the tarsal plate and begin to dissect just deep to the conjunctiva.

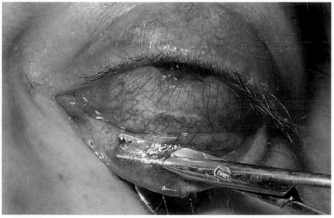

Fig. 11.7a

11.7b

Dissect the conjunctiva off the underlying lower lid retractors as far as the fornix. Cut the tissue just inferior to the fornix (the inferior suspensory ligament of the fornix) to free the fornix.

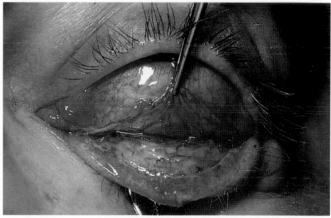

Fig. 11.7b

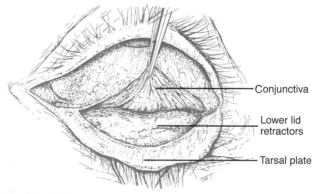

Key diag. 11.7b

- Conjunctiva
- Lower lid retractors
- Tarsal plate

Technique continues overleaf ➔

11:7 **Recession of lower lid retractors** *(Continued)*

11.7c

Incise the lower lid retractors and the septum where they join at the lower border of the tarsal plate to detach them. Dissect them from the orbicularis muscle, lying anteriorly, as far as the fornix. Allow them to retract inferiorly.

11.7d

Prepare a spacer about 15mm transversely and sufficiently wide vertically to achieve as much overcorrection as there was retraction – i.e. for 5mm retraction use a 10mm spacer. Suture one border of the spacer to the recessed retractors using continuous 6/0 plain catgut.

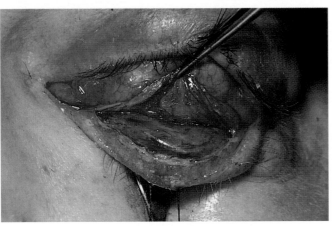

Fig. 11.7c

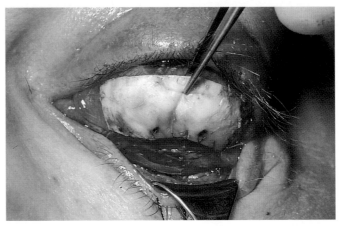

Fig. 11.7d

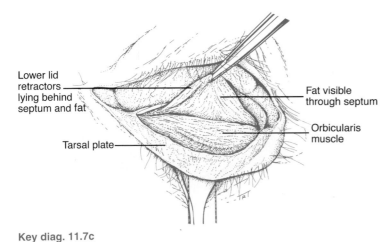

Lower lid retractors lying behind septum and fat

Tarsal plate

Fat visible through septum

Orbicularis muscle

Key diag. 11.7c

Recession of lower lid retractors

11.7e		11.7f

Suture the superior border of the spacer, together with the edge of the conjunctiva, to the inferior border of the tarsal plate.

Pass two or three double-armed 4/0 sutures from the conjunctiva, through the spacer and the full thickness of the lid.

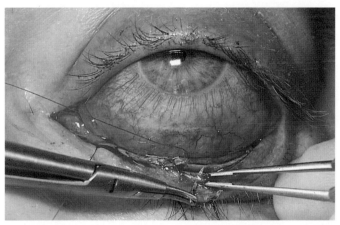

Fig. 11.7e

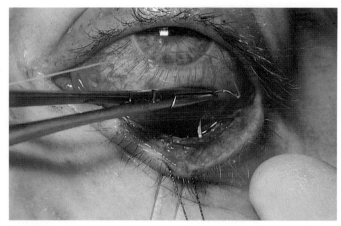

Fig. 11.7f

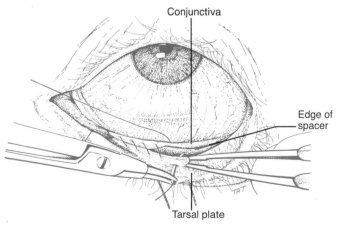

Key diag. 11.7e

Conjunctiva

Edge of spacer

Tarsal plate

Technique continues overleaf →

11:7   Recession of lower lid retractors *(Continued)*

11.7g

Tie the sutures over bolsters on the skin. Tape the traction suture(s) to the forehead for 48 hours. Remove the full – thickness sutures after 7 days.

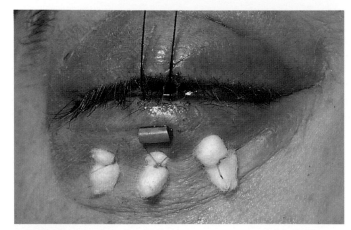

Fig. 11.7g

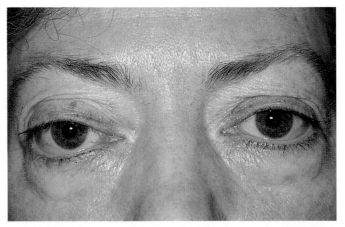

Fig. 11.7 pre

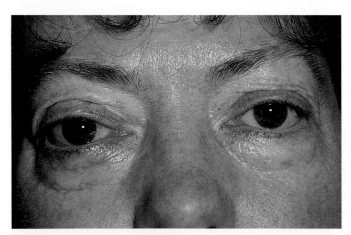

Fig. 11.7 post

Complications and management

Discomfort is frequently a problem if the spacer is not covered with conjunctiva. It usually settles without further surgery as the graft surface becomes epithelialised. All grafts contract but this may be marked in donor sclera. Adequate overcorrection at operation anticipates this.

Other procedures

11:8 Temporary lateral tarsorrhaphy

11.8a

Make an incision approximately 1 mm deep in the grey line of the upper and lower lids from the lateral canthus as far medially as the length of the intended tarsorrhaphy. Excise the lid margin tissues posterior to the incision to a depth of 1 mm or less. Insert double-armed 4/0 non-absorbable mattress sutures which pass through the cut edges and through tarsorrhaphy tubing.

11.8b

Tie the sutures to approximate the lids and leave them in for 2–3 weeks.

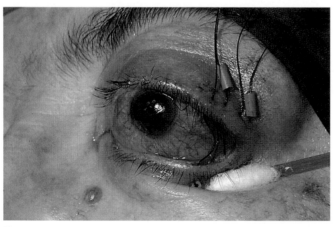

Fig. 11.8a

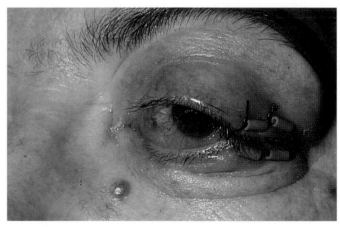

Fig. 11.8b

Complications and management

The tarsorrhaphy may separate in places when the sutures are removed. This can be prevented to some extent by careful approximation of the cut edges. If there is significant tension across the tarsorrhaphy due to lid retraction the upper and lower lid retractors may be cut at the proximal borders of the tarsal plates over the length of the tarsorrhaphy.

11:9 Permanent lateral tarsorrhaphy

This procedure is preferred if a tarsorrhaphy is likely to be needed for more than a few weeks.

11.9a

Make incisions in the grey line in the upper and lower lids from the lateral canthus as far medially as the length of the intended tarsorrhaphy. Deepen the incisions just anterior to the tarsal plates to split the lids into anterior and posterior lamellae as far as the proximal borders of the tarsal plates.

11.9b

Make a vertical cut with scissors through the full height of the upper tarsal plate (arrow) at the medial end of the grey line incision. Make a similar cut in the lower tarsus but now excise the lateral triangle of tarsal plate and conjunctiva which has been created in the lower lid.

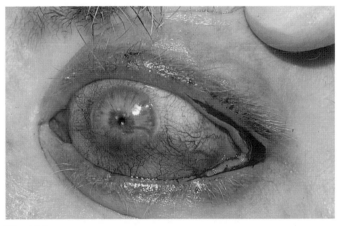

Fig. 11.9a

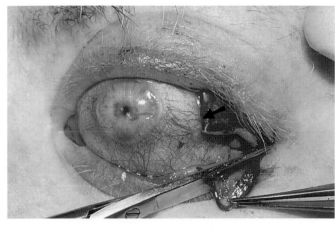

Fig. 11.9b

11.9c

Pass a double-armed 4/0 non-absorbable suture from the apex of the tarsal triangle in the upper lid through the apex of the excised triangular area in the lower lid to emerge on the skin.

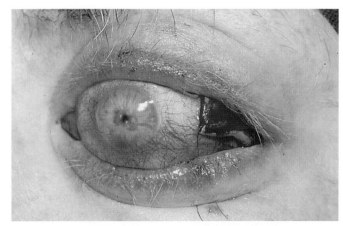

Fig. 11.9c

Technique continues overleaf ➜

11:8 **Temporary lateral tarsorrhaphy** *(Continued)*

11.9d

Tie the suture over a small cotton wool bolster or tarsorrhaphy tubing to draw the triangle of upper lid tarsus into the posterior defect in the lower lid.

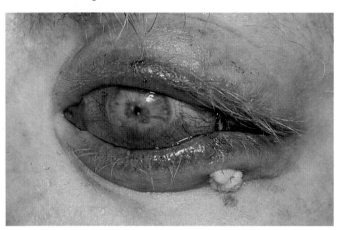

Fig. 11.9d

11.9e

Place mattress sutures to approximate the anterior lamellae of upper and lower lids and to evert the lashes. Remove all sutures at 10 days.

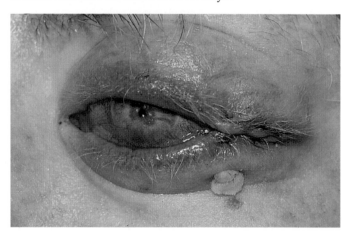

Fig. 11.9e

Complications and management

This type of tarsorraphy rarely breaks down prematurely. Occasionally lashes may be directed posteriorly and cause irritation but this is prevented by careful attention to the anterior lamellar sutures. If posteriorly directed lashes persist cryotherapy to the length of the tarsorrhaphy to clear the lashes may be needed.

Occasionally a fistula between the conjunctiva and the skin may develop and leak tears. Excise the fistula and resuture the lid in layers .

RELATED DISORDERS

Surgical management of thyroid eye disease

Surgery should be postponed until the patient has been euthyroid for at least 6 months unless vision is threatened.

Temporary or permanant lateral tarsorrhaphy (see 11.8, 11.9) may be needed to supplement the procedures recommended below.

Optic nerve compression in the active phase:
— immunosuppression
— steroids, short term
— radiotherapy to orbit
— orbital decompression (see Ch. 18, Sect C)

Diplopia – squint surgery
Upper lid retraction:
— due partly to inferior rectus tethering
— inferior rectus recession
— due to levator muscle infiltration
— retractor recession (11.1–11.4)

Lower lid retraction:
— due to lower lid retractor infiltration
— recession of retractors with a
— spacer (11.7).
— due partly to gross proptosis
— consider orbital decompression

Baggy eyelids:
— consider blepharoplasty (see Ch. 10)

FURTHER READING

Baylis H I et al: Autogenous auricular cartilage grafting for lower eyelid retraction. Ophthalm Plast Reconstr Surg 1: 23; 1985

Dryden R M, Soll D B: The use of scleral transplantation in cicatricial entropion and eyelid retraction. Trans American Acad Ophthalmol Otol 83: 669; 1977

Grove A S: Levator lengthening by marginal myotomy. Arch Opthalmol 98: 1433; 1980

Henderson J W: Relief of eyelid retraction – a surgical procedure. Arch Ophthalmol 74: 205; 1965

Karesh J W, Fabrega MA et al: Polytetraflouroethylene as an interpositonal graft material for the correction of lower eyelid retraction. Opthalmology 96: 419; 1989

Kersten R C, Kulwin DR et al: Management of lower lid retraction with hard palate mucosa grafting. Arch Opthalmol 108: 1339; 1990

Putterman A M, Urist M J: Surgical treatment of upper eyelid retraction. Arch Ophthalmol 87: 401; 1972

Shorr N, Seiff S: The four stages of surgical rehabilitation of the patient with dysthyroid ophthalmopathy. Ophthalmology 93: 476; 1986

Thaller V T, Kaden K, Lane C M, Collin J R O: Thyroid lid surgery. Eye 1: 609; 1987

CHAPTER 12

Evisceration, enucleation, exenteration

Introduction

The emotional distress which frequently accompanies the removal of an eye is reduced considerably by a cosmetic final result. The appearance of the prosthesis will be enhanced and its mobility will be improved if a buried orbital implant is inserted (see Ch. 13) following an evisceration or enucleation.

12:1   Eviscération with removal of the cornea

12.1a

Make a 360 degree conjunctival incision and recess the conjunctiva and Tenon's capsule for a few millimetres from the limbus. Make a 360 degree limbal incision to remove the cornea – start with a scalpel blade or Graefe knife and complete the incision with scissors. Remove the ocular contents with an evisceration spoon and ensure complete removal of all pigmented tissue by careful cleaning of the scleral envelope.

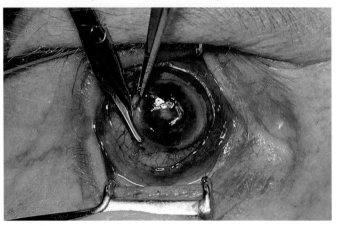

Fig. 12.1a

12.1b

An implant should be inserted and the socket closed if there is no infection. Make two scleral relieving incisions on opposite sides of the limbus to allow the placement of an 18 mm ball implant within the scleral envelope.

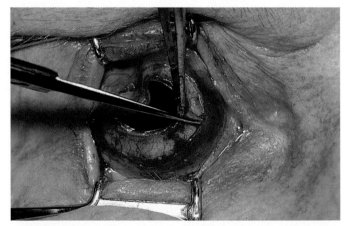

Fig. 12.1b

12.1d

Close Tenon's capsule and the conjunctiva in two layers with 4/0 chromic catgut. Place a conformer in the socket.

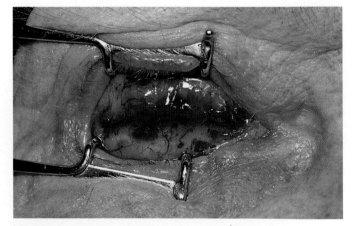

Fig. 12.1d

Alternative procedure

12.1c

Close the sclera over the implant with 6/0 absorbable sutures. If any of the ball is exposed place a patch of donor sclera over the repair (see 13.10).

The cornea may be retained. Make a fornix-based conjunctival flap and a 15mm limbal incision superiorly as for a cataract extraction. Make a 15mm incision in the sclera at 12 o'clock at right angles to the limbal incision. Remove the contents of the eyeball and insert an 18–20mm acrylic ball implant. Suture the limbal incision with an interrupted or continuous fine suture as in cataract surgery. Close the sclera with interrupted 8/0 long-acting absorbable sutures.

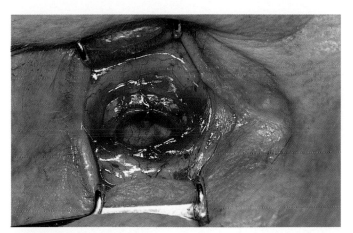

Fig. 12.1c

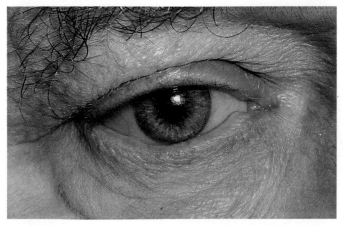

Fig. 12.1 post

Complications and management

Chemosis and lid oedema are common after evisceration. Providing infection does not occur the swelling will settle without treatment.

The risk of sympathetic ophthalmitis in the fellow eye is extremely small but during the follow-up period the fellow eye should be examined.

12.2a

Reflect the conjunctiva from the limbus for 360 degrees. Locate and detach the rectus muscles, placing a suture through each tendon for later identificaiton.

12.2b

Detach the oblique muscles and cut the optic nerve. Take time to achieve complete haemostasis. The inferior oblique muscle may be attached to the lateral rectus muscle, or to an orbital implant between the lateral and inferior rectus muscles, to give added support to an implant.

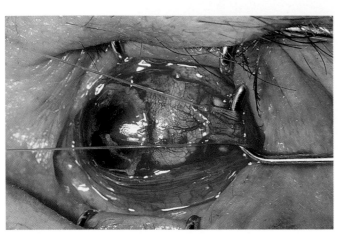

Fig. 12.2a

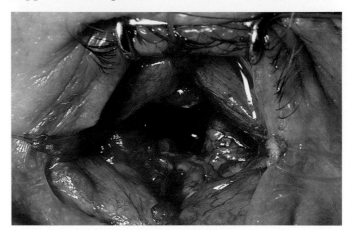

Fig. 12.2b

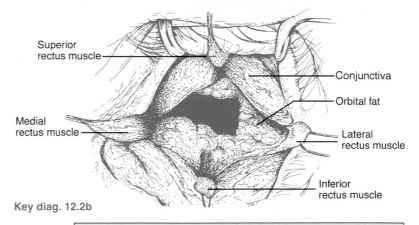

Superior rectus muscle

Medial rectus muscle

Conjunctiva

Orbital fat

Lateral rectus muscle

Inferior rectus muscle

Key diag. 12.2b

12.2c

Insert an appropriate implant (see Ch. 13, Sect. A) unless there is macroscopic tumour extension through the sclera. Close the socket as described in Chapter 13 Sect. A, depending on the implant chosen.
If no implant is inserted leave the rectus muscles free within the orbit and close the conjunctiva with interrupted absorbable sutures.

Complications and management

Haemorrhage from the ophthalmic artery and other vessels close to the orbital apex may be difficult to control and may result in a postoperative orbital haematoma. It may be reduced by the use of a snare to cut the optic nerve. The risk of early extrusion of the orbital implant is increased if a haematoma occurs. Care with haemostasis, if necessary by packing the orbit for 7–10 minutes during surgery, is time well spent.

12:3 Exenteration

This mutilating operation is reserved for tumours of the orbital tissues which cannot be cleared in any other way. It may be necessary to remove bone as well to achieve a satisfactory margin of healthy tissue. If the tumour is posteriorly placed in the orbit, a limited exenteration with preservation of the eyelids may be a safe alternative.

12.3a

Mark the orbital rim, extending the mark slightly anteriorly on the side of the nose to allow removal of the lacrimal sac. Close the eyelids with a suture if necessary.

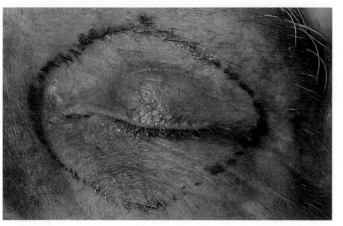

Fig. 12.3a

12.3b

Incise the skin. Cut through the orbicularis muscle to expose the orbital rim periosteum. A cutting diathermy helps to control the bleeding and makes this dissection easier. Incise the periosteum for 360 degrees and reflect the orbital edge with a periosteal elevator.

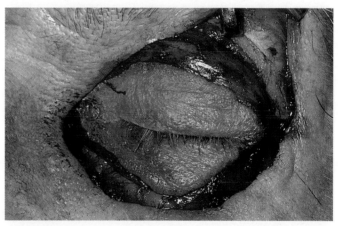

Fig. 12.3b

12.3c

Continue to elevate the periosteum from the orbital walls as far as the apex. Care is needed along the medial wall where the lamina papyracea can be easily fractured.

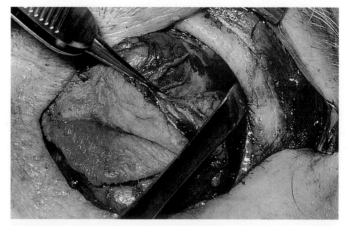

Fig. 12.3c

Technique continues overleaf ➜

12:2   **Enucleation** *(Continued)*

12.3d

Divide the tissues at the apex with curved enucleation scissors or cutting diathermy.

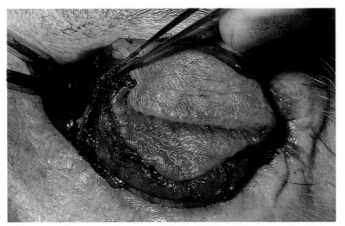

Fig. 12.3d

12.3e

Control haemorrhage from the orbital apex.

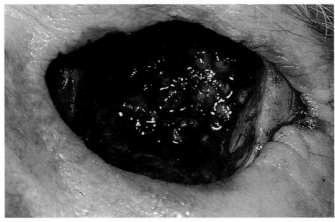

Fig. 12.3e

12.3f

Reduce the skin aperture with sutures placed medially and laterally. Dress the socket with paraffin gauze.

After the first dressing at 48 hours apply twice daily antiseptic dressings such as chlorhexidine or povidone iodine while the socket granulates. The dressings may be reduced to once daily after about 4–6 weeks. Epithelialisation occurs slowly and is usually complete by 3 months.

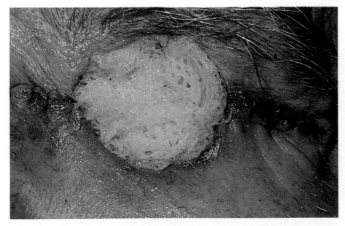

Fig. 12.3f

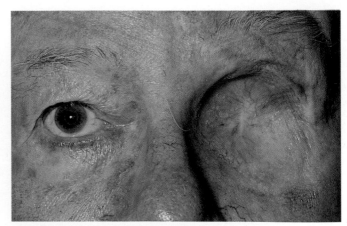

Fig. 12.3 post

Alternative procedures

A   Some or all of the lid skin can be preserved if the tumour is placed posteriorly. Mark the skin to be retained and reflect the skin from the underlying orbicularis muscle as far as the orbital rim. Proceed as described above. At the end fold the lid skin around the orbital rim to line the anterior part of the socket.

B   The socket may be lined with split skin (see 2.10). A deeper socket results than if granulation is allowed to occur. In addition socket hygiene may be more difficult because of skin secretions.

Complications and management

If the lamina papyracea is fractured a communication with the ethmoid air cells can result. There may be some difficulty with healing in that area. Infection of the granulating surfaces may occur, particularly if slough is allowed to build up in the socket. Careful cleansing and the use of antiseptic dressings will control this. A serious infection must be treated with a systemic antibiotic.

FURTHER READING

Bartley G B, Garrity J A, Waller R R et al: Orbital exenteration at the Mayo Clinic. Ophthalmology 96: 468; 1989

Dortzbach R K, Wong J J: Choice of procedure: enucleation, evisceration or prosthetic fitting over globes. Ophthalmology 92: 1249; 1985

Green W R, Maumenee A E, Sanders J E: Sympathetic uveitis following evisceration. Trans Am Acad Ophthalmol Otol 76: 625; 1972

Putterman A M: Orbital exenteration with spontaneous granulation. Arch Ophthalmol 104: 139; 1986

Rudemann A D: Evisceration with retention of the cornea, Am J Ophthalmol 45: 433; 1985

CHAPTER 13

The anophthalmic socket

Introduction

Enucleation and evisceration reduce the volume of the tissues within the orbit. To achieve a cosmetic result this volume must be replaced. A large artificial eye may appear satisfactory at first but with time the lower eyelid will stretch under its weight. The redistribution of orbital fat which follows results in the familiar appearance of the 'postenucleation socket syndrome' – a deep sulcus in the upper eyelid, ptosis or lid retraction, enophthalmos and downward displacement of the eye. This uncosmetic appearance is prevented by the insertion of a buried orbital implant at the time of removal of the eye. If this is not done an implant is often needed at a later date.

Even if a primary implant was inserted at the time of enucleation it may need to be supplemented by another implant if the volume correction is inadequate, or replaced because of exposure or migration.

Finally, contraction of the conjunctival lining of the socket may prevent the artificial eye being worn at all.

Classification: Inadequate volume replacement
Exposed or extruding implant
Contraction of the socket
Other problems – ptosis
– ectropion
– entropion

Primary implants

Choice of operation

As soon as an orbit has been made anophthalmic by enucleation or evisceration of the eye an orbital implant should be inserted. Little extra dissection is required to insert such primary implants and the risk of shallowing the fornices is relatively small. A 'baseball' implant (13.1) provides reliable volume replacement with little late orbital fat reabsorption but a small risk of extrusion. The scleral covering usually contains an acrylic sphere but hydroxyapatite (13.2) is an increasingly popular, although expensive, alternative. The dermofat graft (13.3) loses more volume from reabsorption during the first 6–9 months but has a very low extrusion rate. Because the conjunctiva is sutured to the edges of tie of a dermofat graft, the fornices are shallowed less than with other implants.

13:1   Primary 'baseball' implant

The 'baseball' implant is an acrylic sphere wrapped in donor sclera. It gives excellent volume replacement and the rectus muscles are attached to it to improve motility. Use a whole donor sclera prepared as described in 2.15. An alternative to donor sclera which has given similar results is Mersilene mesh.

13.1a

Choose a plastic ball which just fits into the orbit. Its overal size will be slightly increased by the scleral envelope. Too small an implant will leave space unfilled. Too large an implant may make the fitting of a prosthesis difficult. Close the sclera (or other covering) over the ball using 6/0 long-acting absorbable sutures.

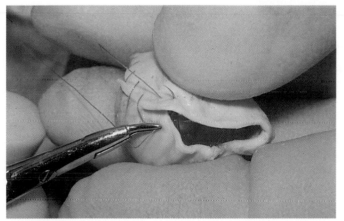

Fig. 13.1a A

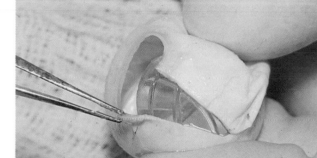

Fig. 13.1a B

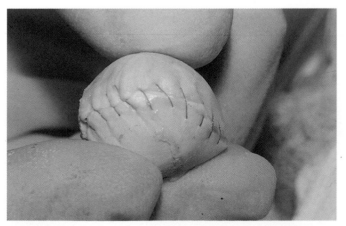

Fig. 13.1a C

13.1b

Open posterior Tenon's capsule by spreading with scissors to expose the orbital fat.

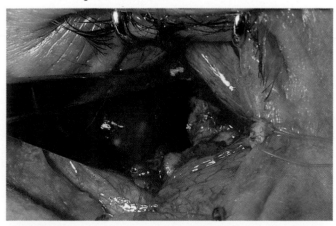

Fig. 13.1b

Technique continues overleaf →

13:1 | **Primary 'baseball' implant** *(Continued)*

13.1c

Place the implant, with the sutures posteriorly, into the muscle cone. Pass double-armed 4/0 chromic catgut sutures through the tendons of the four rectus muscles. Use these sutures to attach the rectus muscles to the sclera in their normal orientation and about 1 cm posterior to the anterior pole of the implant.

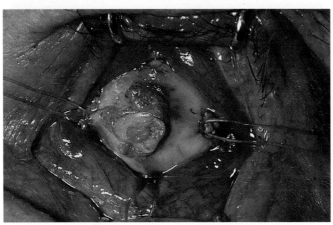

Fig. 13.1c

13.1d

Pass the two needles of each suture through Tenon's capsule and the conjuctiva into the adjacent fornix taking care that when these sutures are tied Tenon's capsule and the conjunctiva can be closed over the implant without tension. Take care also not to place the sutures too far peripherally, especially in the lower fornix, or the fornices may be shallowed.

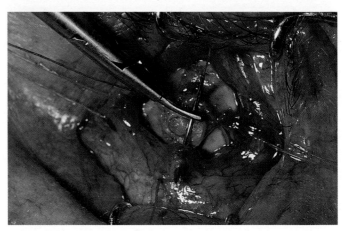

Fig. 13.1d

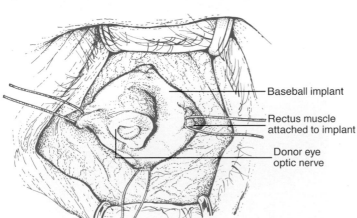

Baseball implant

Rectus muscle attached to implant

Donor eye optic nerve

Key diag. 13.1c

13.1e

13.1e Tie the fornix sutures (arrow). Close Tenon's capsule and the conjunctiva, without tension, in two layers with 4/0 chromic catgut.

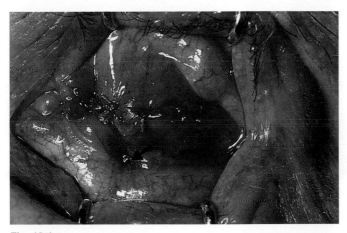

Fig. 13.1e

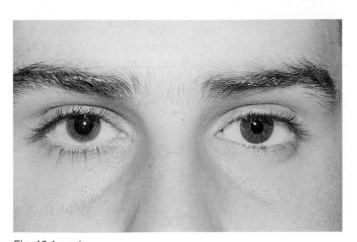

Fig. 13.1 post

Complications and management

The fornices, especially the lower fornix, may be shallowed if there is inadequate conjunctiva or if the closure over the implant draws too much conjunctiva out of the fornices. If a prosthesis cannot be fitted or worn satisfactorily deepen the fornix with oral mucosa (13.12).

Exposure of the implant may lead to extrusion if it is not dealt with promptly (13.10). If extrusion occurs allow the socket to heal and reassess with a view to a secondary implant (Sect. B). Migration of the implant, often inferiorly and laterally, makes the fitting of a satisfactory prosthesis difficult. Remove the migrated implant and insert a secondary implant in the correct position within the muscle cone.

13.2a

Hydroxyapatite binds to the tissues of the orbit so plastic balls are used to assess the size of implant needed. Soak the appropriate hydroxyapatite ball in gentamicin and place it into a donor sclera (or other covering material). Close the sclera around the hydroxyapatite and suture it, leaving a gap, this will be the posterior aspect of the implant. Mark and cut out small rectangular windows through the sclera about 5 mm from the anterior pole of the implant for the insertions of the rectus muscles. A fifth window is cut for the inferior oblique muscle.

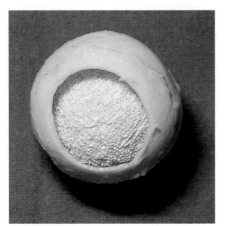

Fig. 13.2a A

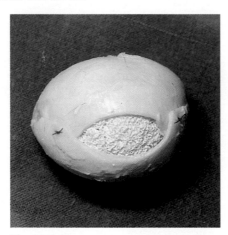

Fig. 13.2a B

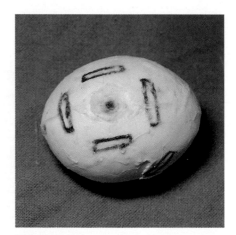

Fig. 13.2a C

13.2d

Close Tenon's capsule and the conjunctiva in two layers with 6/0 absorbable sutures. Place a conformer.

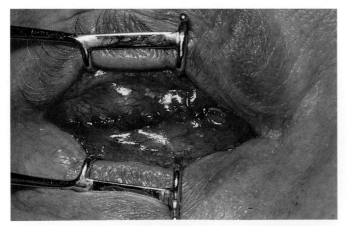

Fig. 13.2d

At approximately 6 months postoperatively a peg may be inserted into the implant for articulation with the prosthesis. The implant must be fully vascularised and this is confirmed with a gallium-67 bone scan. Many patients decide against this second procedure because of satisfactory cosmesis without it. The techniques for peg insertion and fitting a prosthesis will not be described but see 'Further reading'.

Complications and management

As for the baseball implant.

In addition, the vascularisation of the hydroxyapatite may be inadequate and drilling the implant to insert a peg may result in exposure or extrusion of the implant.

13.2b

Attach double-armed 4/0 absorbable sutures to the muscle insertions and pass both needles through the anterior edges of the scleral windows to draw the insertions into the windows.

13.2c

Having inserted the muscles into the scleral windows check that Tenon's capsule and the conjunctiva can be closed over the implant without tension.

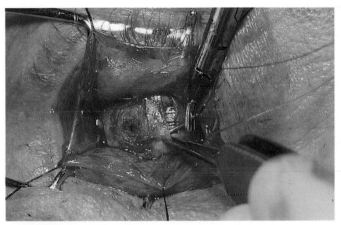

Fig. 13.2b

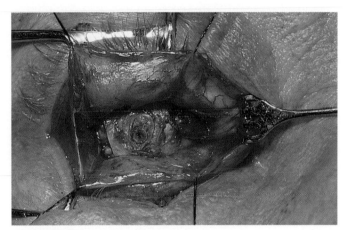

Fig. 13.2c

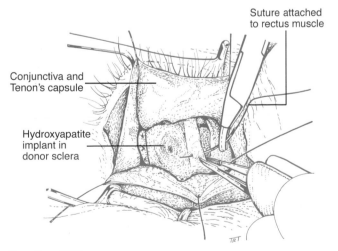

Suture attached
to rectus muscle

Conjunctiva and
Tenon's capsule

Hydroxyapatite
implant in
donor sclera

Key diag. 13.2b

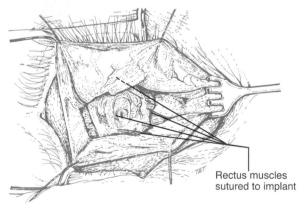

Rectus muscles
sutured to implant

Key diag. 13.2c

13:3 | Primary dermofat graft

General anaesthesia is used and the patient is placed in the left lateral position.

13.3a

Mark a sickle-shaped ellipse approximately 6 cm in its long axis and 2.5 cm across, convex posteriorly, in the middle third of the buttock and following the curve of the buttock. Incise the epidermis and inject saline intradermally. Carefully remove the epidermis with a curved scalpel blade (Bard Parker no. 10 or 15) to the depth of a moderate split skin graft. The skin removed should not be paper thin and translucent but moderately opaque leaving multiple focal haemorrhages and scattered small foci of exposed fat on the donor site. Large globules of exposed fat indicate too deep a dissection.

13.3b

Deepen the incision vertically at the edge of the ellipse to about 2.5 cm into the underlying fat.

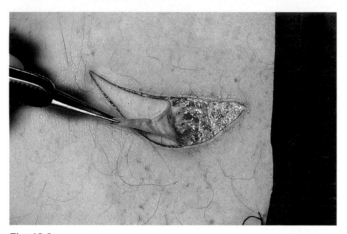

Fig. 13.3a

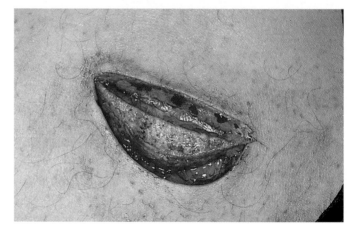

Fig. 13.3b

13.3c

Gently remove the dermofat graft. (*Note* – the sciatic nerve is approximately halfway between the greater trochanter of the femur and the ischial tuberosity, deep to the lower part of the gluteus maximus muscle, so it is relatively well protected during this operation).

13.3d

Place the dermofat graft into the socket with the dermis anteriorly. The fat should slightly 'overfill' the socket to allow for some absorption.

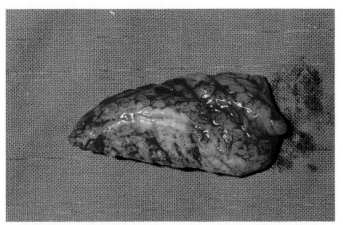

Fig. 13.3c

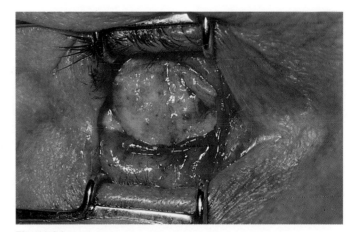

Fig. 13.3d

Close the defect with several layers of 4/0 chromic catgut to close the fat and subcutaneous tissues and interrupted 4/0 silk to the skin. Use a supporting Elastoplast dressing for about 5 days and remove the sutures in 10 days.

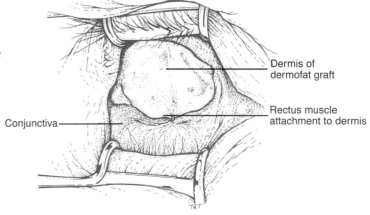

Dermis of dermofat graft

Rectus muscle attachment to dermis

Conjunctiva

Key diag. 13.3d

Technique continues overleaf ➔

13:3 **Primary dermofat graft** *(Continued)*

13.3e,f

Trim the graft if necessary. Suture the four rectus muscles to the edge of the dermis with 6/0 chromic catgut. The conjunctiva does not need to cover the whole graft but it should be sutured to its anterior surface to cover the edge using a 6/0 absorbable suture.

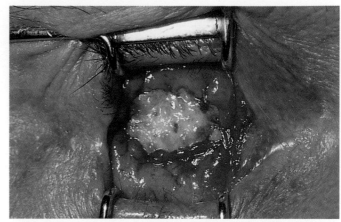

Fig. 13.3e

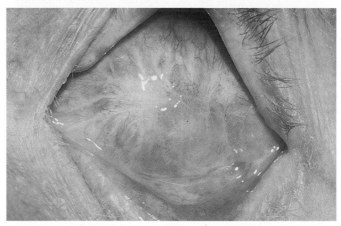

Fig. 13.3f Epithelialisation occurs within a month or so.

Complications and management

The fat in the graft reduces in volume during the first 6–12 months. The absorption is greater when this graft is used as a secondary implant. However, the advantage to the fornices is not lost (see Choice of Operation).

If the split thickness skin removed from the surface of the graft is too thick fat will be visible and epithelialisation may be delayed. Complete cover will eventually be achieved.

If the skin removed is too thin adnexal remnants may lead to keratinisation and the growth of hairs on the surface of the graft. These result in discomfort as soon as a prosthesis is fitted. If they persist cryotherapy as a double freeze-thaw to −20°C will usually eliminate hair growth but keratinised areas may need to be removed surgically.

If the edge of the graft separates from the host conjunctiva fat will prolapse. If this is small wait for epithelialisation to occur. If the prolapse is large resuture the edge of the graft. Sweat gland remnants or conjunctival ingrowth can lead to cyst formation.

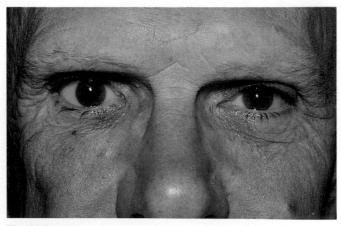

Fig. 13.3 post

Secondary implants

Choice of operation

If an anophthalmic socket has healed without an implant or with an inadequate implant, or if the implant has extruded, a secondary implant is required. An inadequate implant, whether primary or secondary, in the muscle cone may be supplemented by an orbital floor implant (13.7, 13.8).

If the fornices are obviously shallow before an implant is inserted they must be reconstructed (13.12, 13.13) before an implant is inserted or at the same time. If the fornices are deep a baseball implant (13.4), or an alternative solid implant such as a hydroxyapatite implant (13.5), is suitable. If the fornices are shallowed but do not require extra mucosa a dermofat graft (13.6) is preferred with the conjunctiva sutured to the edge of the graft. The alternative is a solid implant with fornix reconstruction.

If more than one implant extrusion has occurred from a socket a dermofat graft may be retained better than a solid implant.

13:4 Secondary baseball implant

As a secondary implant the baseball implant has all the advantages of a primary baseball implant. It may, however, further reduce the depth of an already shallow fornix. The donor sclera encloses an acrylic ball.

13.4a

Make a horizontal incision with scissors across the centre of the socket – the original line of closure of the conjunctiva is a good guide – and deepen it through Tenon's capsule until orbital fat is exposed.

13.4b

Enlarge the access to the intraconal space by spreading with scissors.

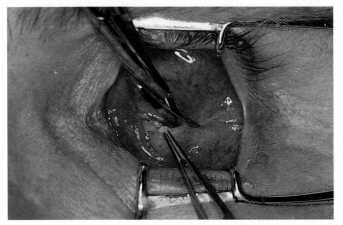

Fig. 13.4a

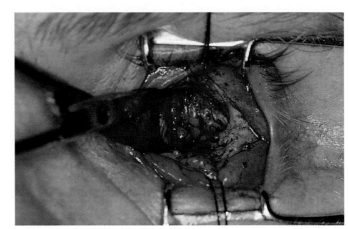

Fig. 13.4b

13.4c

If an existing implant is to be removed try to identify and preserve the rectus muscles if attached. If no implant is in situ attempt to dissect out the four rectus muscles.

13.4d

Prepare the implant and attach the rectus muscles, if found, as described above (13.1c,d). If the muscles have not been found attach the double-armed sutures to the baseball implant as in 13.1c,d and pass them directly through Tenon's capsule and conjunctiva to the fornices. It is most important that the implant is inserted above and not below the inferior rectus muscle or the lower lid will not move due to disruption of the lower lid retractors.

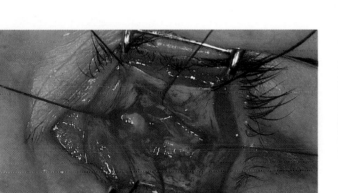

Fig. 13.4c

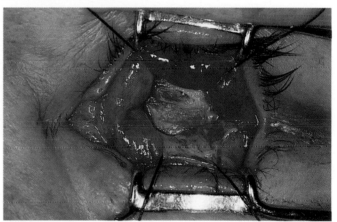

Fig. 13.4d

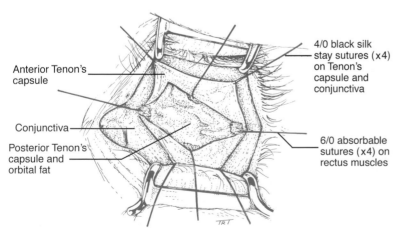

Anterior Tenon's capsule

Conjunctiva

Posterior Tenon's capsule and orbital fat

4/0 black silk stay sutures (x4) on Tenon's capsule and conjunctiva

6/0 absorbable sutures (x4) on rectus muscles

Key diag. 13.4c

Technique continues overleaf →

13:4 Secondary baseball implant

13.4e

Tie the fornix sutures and close Tenon's capsule and the conjunctiva in two layers (see 13.1e). Fit a conformer.

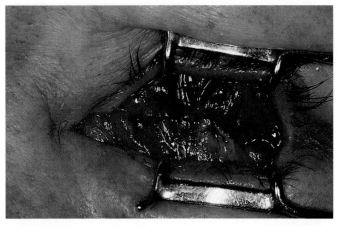

Fig. 13.4e

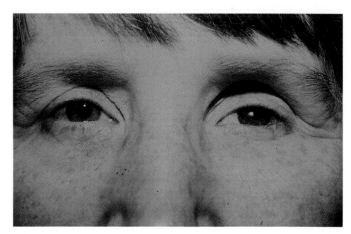

Fig 13.4 pre

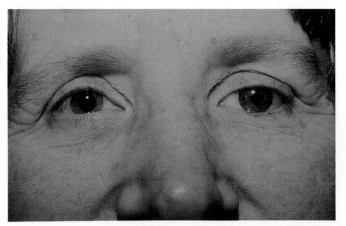

Fig. 13.4 post

Complications and management

As for primary baseball implant. Note also the importance of placing the implant within the muscle cone and not below the inferior rectus muscle.

13:5 Secondary hydroxyapatite implant

13.5a

Prepare the socket (see 13.4a–c). Use plastic balls to assess the size of hydroxyapatite required. The implant may be inserted into the muscle cone without a covering. This enhances vascularisation. Because hydroxyapatite tends to bind to the tissues during surgery, it is easier to insert it into the muscle cone wrapped in two half-sheets of fine polythene which meet at the posterior pole of the implant. These can be gently eased out once the implant is in place.

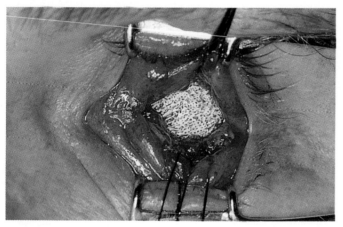

Fig. 13.5a

13.5b

Close Tenon's capsule, without tension, over the implant.

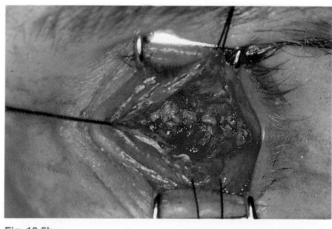

Fig. 13.5b

13.5c

If there is any doubt about the security of the tissues anterior to the implant it is safer to insert a scleral patch anterior to Tenon's capsule (see 13.10), before closing the conjunctiva.

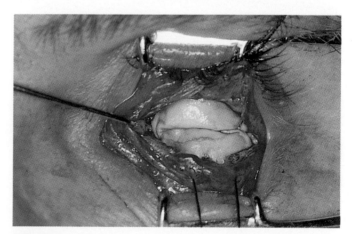

Fig. 13.5c

Technique continues overleaf →

Secondary hydroxyapatite implant

13:6 Secondary dermofat graft

13.5d

Close the conjunctiva with 6/0 absorbable sutures.

Take a dermofat graft (see 13.3). If an implant has been removed the capsule must be excised to allow vascularisation of the graft. The graft should be large enough just to 'overfill' the available space in the orbit to allow for reabsorption which is usually more marked than with a primary implant. Suture the rectus muscles and conjunctiva as for a primary dermofat graft.

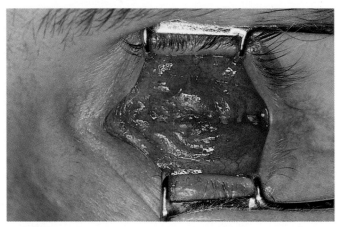

Fig. 13.5d

A peg may be inserted at about 6 months (see comment 13.2d).

Complications and management

As for primary hydroxyapatite implants.

Complications and management

As for primary dermofat grafts but loss of volume during the first 6 months is greater than primary grafts.

13:7   Subperiosteal orbital floor implant – subciliary approach

13.7a

Make an incision in the skin 1–2 mm below the lash line and extend it laterally then downwards at the lateral canthus.

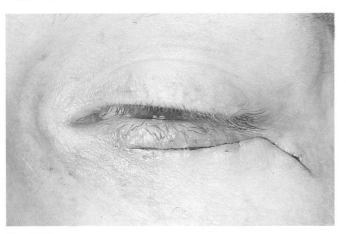

Fig. 13.7a

13.7b

Turn down the flap of skin and orbicularis to expose the inferior orbital rim, taking care not to damage the orbital septum lying immediately deep to orbicularis.

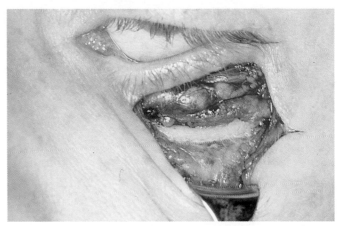

Fig. 13.7b

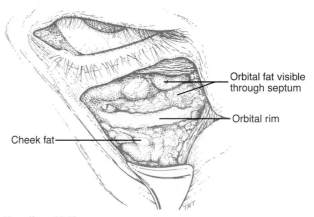

Orbital fat visible through septum

Orbital rim

Cheek fat

Key diag. 13.7b

Technique continues overleaf →

13:7 Subperiosteal orbital floor implant – subciliary approach *(Continued)*

13.7c

Incise the periosteum along the inferior orbital rim. Using a small periosteal elevator raise the periosteum either side of the incision to expose the bony rim. Extend the dissection posteriorly to expose the whole of the orbital floor.

13.7d

Assess the available space in the floor of the orbit and cut an implant, from silicone sheet 2–4mm thick, to fit it. Pre-fashioned implants are available but a 'tailor-made' implant cut at operation from a block of silicone allows an exact fit to the floor of the orbit.

Drill two pairs of holes through the orbital rim in preparation for wires to fix the implant.

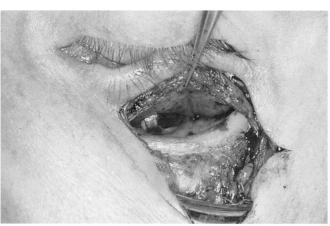

Fig. 13.7c

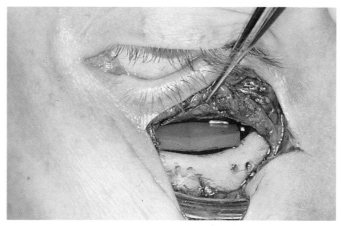

Fig. 13.7d

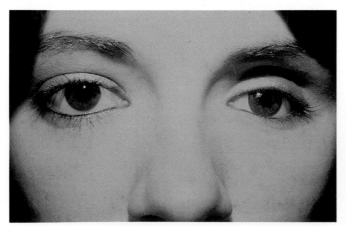

Fig. 13.7 pre

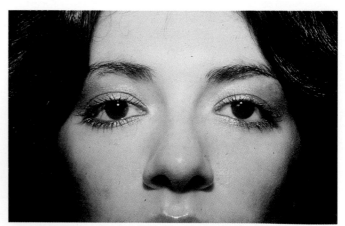

Fig. 13.7 post

Subperiosteal orbital floor implant – subciliary approach

13.7e

Drill matching pairs of holes in the implant. Wire the implant to the orbital rim using fine stainless steel wire.

13.7f

Close the periosteum with a 4/0 absorbable suture. Place a suture at the angle of the incision. Use buried 6/0 long-acting absorbable sutures to close the muscle. Close the skin incision with 6/0 sutures.

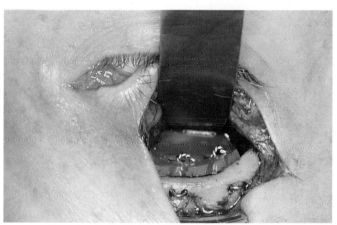

Fig. 13.7e

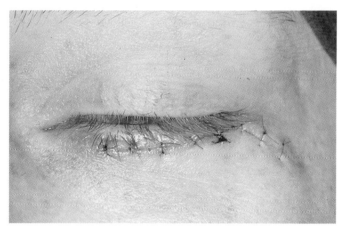

Fig. 13.7f

Complications and management

Too small an implant to correct the volume deficit is common. The profile of the implant should be thicker posteriorly to push the existing implant upwards and forwards.

The implanted silicone may migrate forwards causing a palpable mass in the lower lid. This is usually eliminated by wiring a single-piece implant to the orbital rim. If migration occurs trim the anterior face of the implant.

If the lower fornix is distorted or shallowed by the anterior edge of the implant it may be necessary to revise the implant to allow a prosthesis to be fitted.

13:8 Subperiosteal orbital floor implant – McCord approach

13.8a

Make an oblique cut with scissors through the lid from the lateral canthus down and laterally to the orbital rim.

13.8b

Dissect by spreading scissors to expose the lateral 1.5 cm of the inferior orbital rim. Incise the periosteum and free it with a small periosteal elevator to expose the floor of the orbit. Take care to leave the remaining periosteum intact along the inferior orbital rim. This will prevent forward movement of the implant. Lift the periosteum from the floor of the orbit as far as the apex.

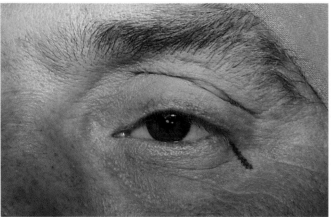

Fig. 13.8a

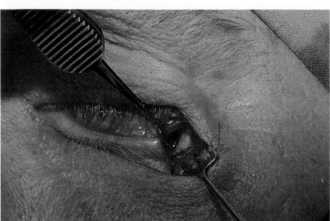

Fig. 13.8b

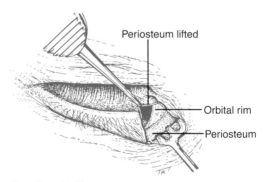

Key diag. 13.8b

Subperiosteal orbital floor implant – McCord approach

13.8c

Cut a suitable implant from a silicone block (see 13.7d), estimating its size and shape. Cut the implant into pieces small enough to be inserted through the periosteal incision.

13.8d

Insert the strips of silicone. Arrange the pieces as far as possible to reform the shape of the implant in the floor of the orbit. The implant will not be wired so no drill holes are needed in the orbital rim.

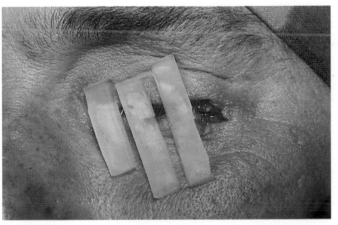

Fig. 13.8c

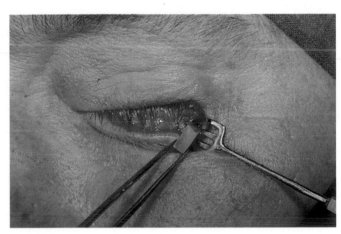

Fig 13.8d

13.8e

Close the periosteum with a 4/0 absorbable suture. Place a plastic conformer, or the patient's artificial eye, in the socket and estimate the degree of lid laxity, if any, by pulling the lid laterally. Leaving a strip of

tarsus intact remove the excess lateral skin, muscle and conjunctiva. Attach the tarsal strip to the periosteum of the lateral orbital rim with a 6/0 absorbable suture.

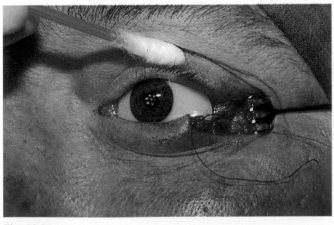

Fig. 13.8e

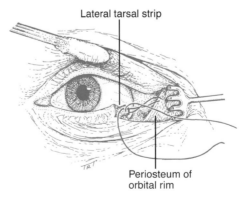

Key diag. 13.8e

Technique continues overleaf ➜

13:8   Subperiosteal orbital floor implant – McCord approach *(Continued)*

13.8f

Take care to close the orbicularis and skin in two layers or a fistula through the lid may result.

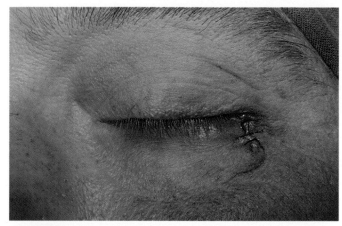

Fig. 13.8f

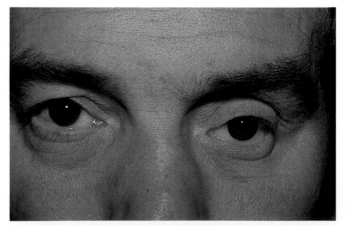

Fig. 13.8 pre

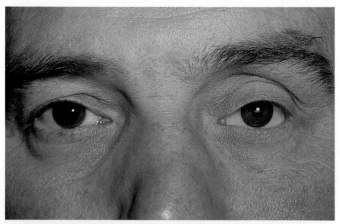

Figs. 13.8 post Ptosis to be corrected. Persistent deep upper lid sulcus may need a dermofat graft, (13.9).

Complications and management

As for 13.7. The strips of unwired silicone may migrate forward and be palpable through the lower lid. Trim the anterior edges if necessary.

13:9 Dermofat graft to the superior sulcus

If a deep superior sulcus persists in the upper lid despite apparently adequate volume replacement in the orbit, a dermofat graft may be used to fill out the sulcus.

13.9a

Take a dermofat graft (see 13.3). The size of graft needed for the superior sulcus is smaller than for the intraconal space.

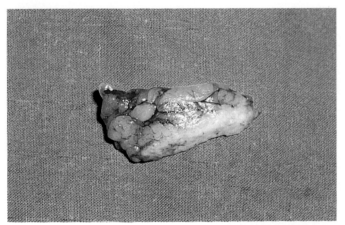

Fig. 13.9a

13.9b

Make a skin crease incision in the upper lid and expose the orbital septum (see 9.2). Open the septum to expose the preaponeurotic fat (see 9.2b–d).

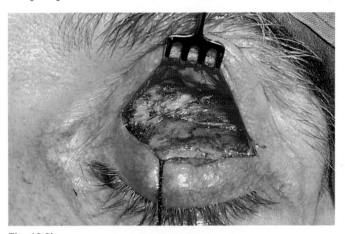

Fig. 13.9b

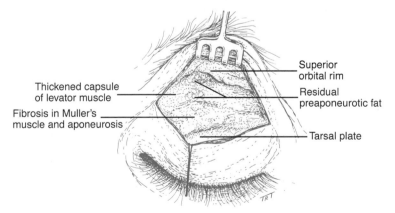

Thickened capsule of levator muscle

Fibrosis in Muller's muscle and aponeurosis

Superior orbital rim

Residual preaponeurotic fat

Tarsal plate

Key diag. 13.9b

Technique continues overleaf →

13:9 **Dermofat graft to the superior sulcus** *(Continued)*

13.9c

Trim the graft to fit into the preaponeurotic space with some excess to allow for graft reabsorption. Suture the dermis to the periosteum of the orbital roof, just posterior to the orbital rim, with interrupted 6/0 absorbable sutures.

13.9d

Close the skin with 6/0 interrupted sutures taking deep bites into the anterior surface of the levator aponeurosis to create a skin crease. Remove the sutures in 2 weeks or allow to absorb.

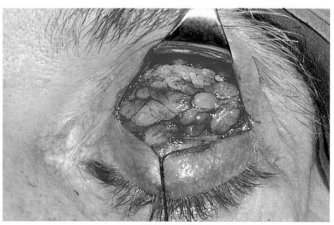

Fig. 13.9c

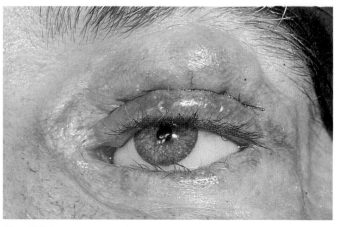

Fig. 13.9d

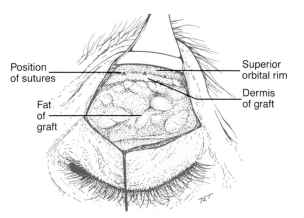

Position of sutures
Superior orbital rim
Fat of graft
Dermis of graft

Key diag. 13.9c

Dermofat graft to the superior sulcus

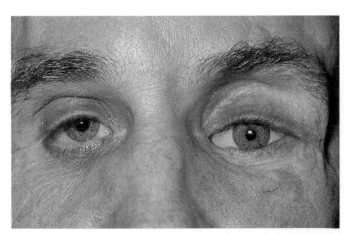 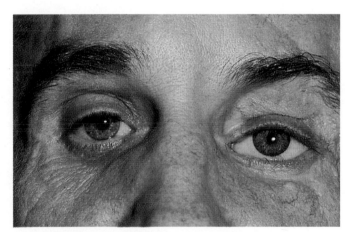

Figs 13.9 Pre, Post Severe trauma to left orbital bones and soft tissues. Prosthesis to be modified.

Complications and management

The graft should be oversized in anticipation of some fat reabsorption. This causes a ptosis in the early weeks after surgery. If the volume of fat remains too large after 12 months it may be reduced through a skin crease incision. If too much fat volume is lost the dermofat graft may be repeated.

Exposed and extruding orbital implants

13:10 Scleral patch

13.10a

Early exposure of an implant (arrow) may be closed with a patch of donor sclera. If the implant has been exposed for more than a month it is safer to remove it with its capsule and insert a secondary implant.

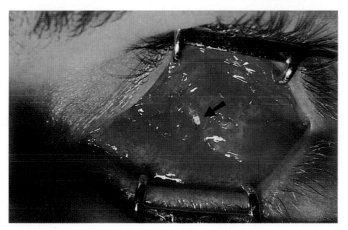

Fig. 13.10a

13.10b

Incise the conjunctiva horizontally and dissect it free from the underlying Tenon's capsule as far as the fornices in all directions. This can be a difficult dissection through scarred tissue and Tenon's capsule may not be dissected out intact.

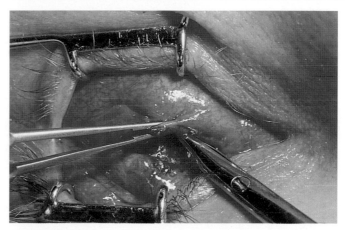

Fig. 13.10b

13.10c

Cut a patch of donor sclera (see 2.15) large enough to extend easily out to the fornices.

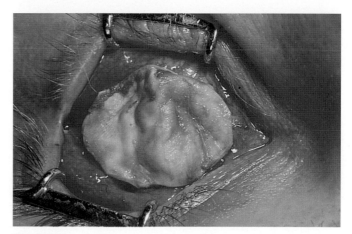

Fig. 13.10c

Technique continues overleaf →

13:10 **Scleral patch** *(Continued)*

13.10d

Place the scleral patch between Tenon's capsule and the conjunctiva. Fix the patch to Tenon's capsule with interrupted 6/0 absorbable sutures around its edge. Check that the conjunctiva can close without tension. If not, extend the dissection further into the fornices to mobilise it.

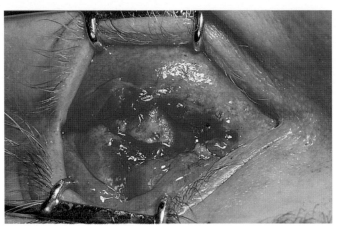

Fig. 13.10d

13.10e

Close the conjunctiva over the patch and fit a conformer in the socket.

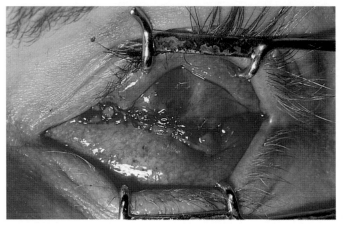

Fig. 13.10e

Complications and management

The exposed implant may still extrude despite this attempt to cover it. If it becomes exposed despite the scleral patch, remove it and replace it with a secondary implant.

Contracting socket

Choice of operation

The lower fornix usually contracts first. Providing the conjunctiva is still elastic and can be stretched easily down into the lower fornix, sutures placed to maintain the depth (13.11) may be all that is required. If marked contraction of the conjunctiva of the socket is established extra mucosa must be inserted (13.12, 13.13)

13:11 Fornix deepening sutures

13.11a

Using a large needle with an eye pass three 4/0 nylon sutures through a conformer of silicone rod or gutter.

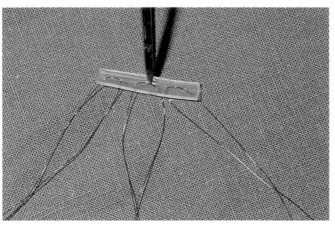

Fig. 13.11a

13.11b

Pass the needles from the depths of the fornix out to the skin, being careful to include the periosteum of the inferior orbital rim.

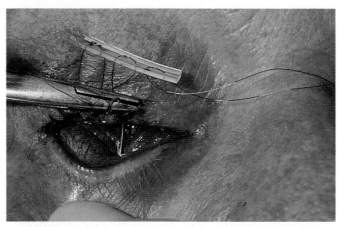

Fig. 13.11b

13.11e

Aim to deepen the fornix without distorting the position of the lower lid.

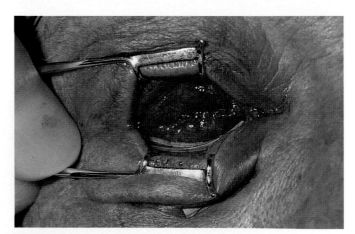

Fig. 13.11e

Remove the sutures at 3 weeks.

Fornix deepening sutures

13.11c

Pull on the sutures to position the conformer in the fornix.

13.11d

Finally pass each suture through a second conformer on the skin, tighten and tie them. (See also 13.12d).

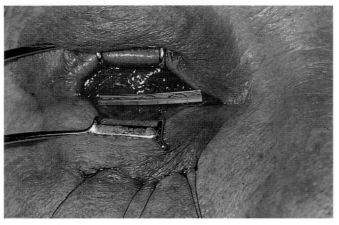

Fig. 13.11c

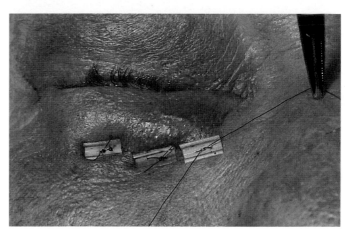

Fig. 13.11d

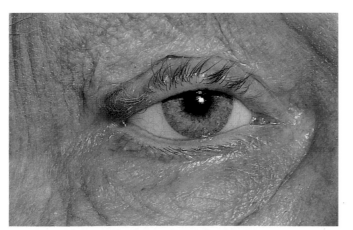

Fig. 13.11 post

Complications and management

Gross distortion of the lower lid will be obvious at surgery and is usually due to incorrect positioning of the sutures in the fornix or on the skin. Reposition them.

Haemorrhage is common and a haematoma may form. It does not usually need to be evacuated.

Alt

13:

Incis
close
it fro
deep
upp
muc
con
thro
upp

CHAPTER 14

Eyelid reconstruction – introduction

Normal eyelids have an anterior covering layer and a posterior supporting layer with a lining. Whenever possible this combination of the two most important layers should be restored. At least one of the two layers must have a blood supply. A free graft placed on another free graft will fail.

Partial thickness defects usually involve only the anterior covering layer. Chapter 15 describes the commonly used methods of reconstructing this anterior layer. If a full thickness defect of the lid has to be reconstructed a posterior supporting layer is also needed. Chapter 16 describes techniques of providing this layer. An alternative approach is to reconstruct a full thickness defect with a full thickness flap which includes both anterior and posterior layers. Chapter 17 describes frequently used full thickness techniques.

Choice of operation

Small eyelid defects, up to one-quarter of the lid length or up to one-third in elderly patients, can usually be closed directly (see 2.6) without the need for 'reconstruction' using tissues from elsewhere. Other techniques, described below, allow even larger defects to the closed directly. These are lateral cantholysis (14.1), the semicircular skin flap (14.2) and the McGregor cheek flap (14.3).

14:1 Lateral cantholysis

This technique allows direct closure of most upper or lower lid defects up to one-third of the lid length.

14.1a

Make a horizontal cut from the lateral canthus to the orbital rim.

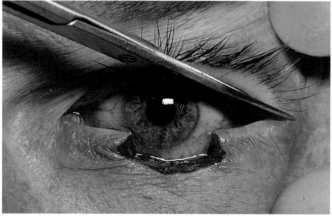

Fig. 14.1a

14.1b

Pull the lid medially to put the appropriate limb of the lateral canthal tendon on stretch. It can now be felt as a tight band just posterior to the orbicularis muscle. Expose this limb of the tendon by spreading scissors either side of it.

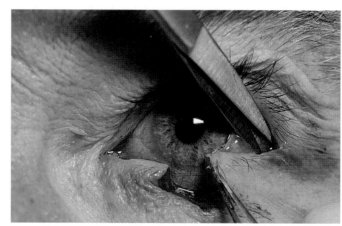

Fig. 14.1b

14.1d

Close the lid defect in the usual way (see 2.6). Close the lateral wound, skin to conjunctiva and skin to skin, with 6/0 sutures.

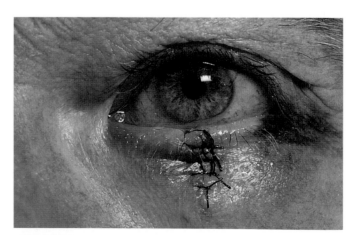

Fig. 14.1d

14.1c

Cut this limb of the tendon.

If the defect cannot be closed without undue tension the orbital septum between the lateral tarsal fragment and the inferior orbital rim must be cut to allow the lateral tissues to move further medially. To do this grasp the medial cut end of the tendon and pull it laterally and slightly upwards to put the septum on stretch. Gently introduce scissors between the orbicularis muscle and the conjunctiva along the inferior orbital rim and cut the septum as far medially as necessary to allow closure of the lid. With each cut into the septum the lid will be felt to 'give' and become more mobile.

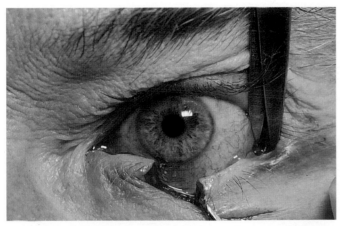

Fig. 14.1c

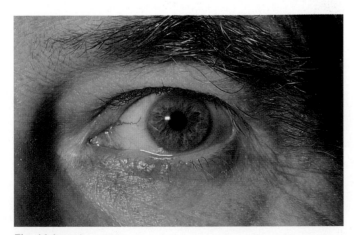

Fig. 14.1 post

Complications and management

A shallow depression in the lateral lid margin is due to poor support for the anterior lamella. To avoid this take care that the initial incision (14.1a) does not stray downwards into the skin of the lower lid laterally.

14:2 Semicircular flap (Tenzel)

This technique allows direct closure of upper or lower lid defects up to about one-half of the lid length.

14.2a

Mark the semicircular flap approximately 22 mm in the vertical and 18 mm in the horizontal direction. Begin the mark as a lateral continuation of the line of the lid to be reconstructed. Continue more steeply upwards (for reconstruction of the lower lid) or downwards (for reconstruction of the upper lid), curving the line to achieve the correct dimensions. Finish level with the canthus and no further lateral than the end of the eyebrow.

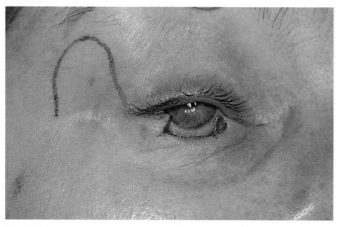

Fig. 14.2a

14.2b

Make an incision along the mark and undermine the flap in the plane just deep to orbicularis muscle. Do not dissect lateral to the orbital rim. Reflect the flap to expose the lateral canthus.

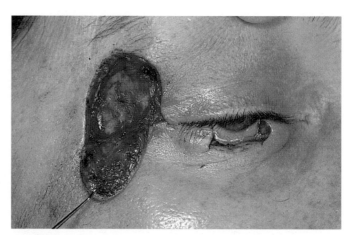

Fig. 14.2b

14.2e

Close the edge of the flap in two layers with 6/0 catgut and a 6/0 non-absorbable suture to the skin. Remove the surface sutures at 5 days.

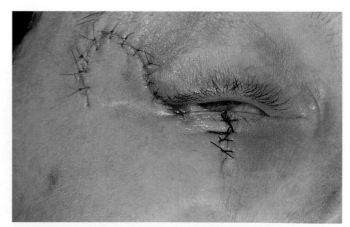

Fig. 14.2e

14.2c

Cut the appropriate limb of the lateral canthal tendon (arrow). For closure of a lower lid defect free the septum (see 14.1c).

14.2d

Close the eyelid defect in the usual way (see 2.6). Pull the lid gently laterally to remove any horizontal lid laxity. Support the flap with a 4/0 non-absorbable suture (arrow) to the deep tissues. Where the flap edge crosses the lateral canthus fix it to the oppisite limb of the lateral canthal tendon with a 4/0 long-acting absorbable suture to create a new canthus.

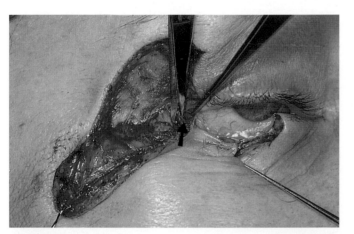

Fig. 14.2c

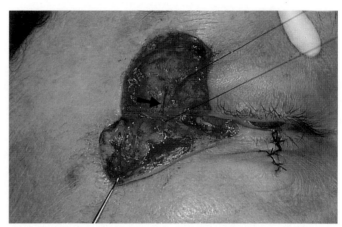

Fig. 14.2d

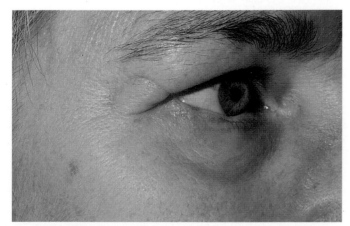

Fig. 14.2 post

Complications and management

It is important that the line of incision from the lateral canthus is not horizontal but a continuation of the line of the lid to be reconstructed. If this is not done a shallow depression will appear in the lateral part of the reconstructed lid margin.

14:3 McGregor cheek flap

This flap utilises a Z-plasty which helps to avoid a dog-ear in the superior edge of the wound and partly hides the scar by breaking the line.

14.3a

Mark an incision from the lateral canthus towards the ear with a gentle curve convex upward (for the lower lid) or downward (for the upper lid). Mark a Z with the stem along the main incision, placing the more lateral limb of the Z on the same side of the main incision as the lid to be reconstructed,

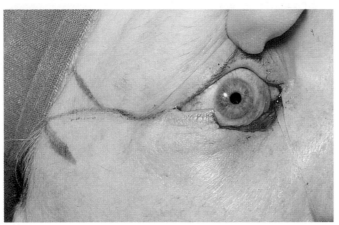

Fig. 14.3a

14.3b

Reflect the flaps keeping deep to the orbicularis muscle while medial to the orbital rim. Dissect superficial to orbicularis lateral to the orbital rim. Undermine beyond the flaps. Cut the appropriate limb of the lateral canthal tendon and mobilise the lateral part of the lid (see 14.1c). Close the defect in the lid (see 2.6). Transpose the flaps in the usual way (see 2.20).

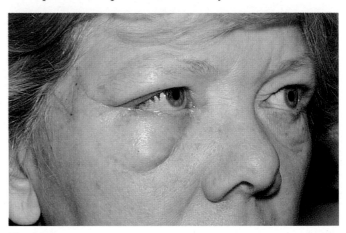

Fig. 14.3b

Complications and management

Oedema in the lid is common because the lymphatic drainage is interrupted when the flaps are cut. It disappears after several weeks.

FURTHER READING

Mustarde J C: Repair and reconstruction in the orbital region, 3rd edn. Churchill Livingstone, Edinburgh; 1991

Tenzel R R: Reconstruction of the central one half of an eyelid. Arch Ophthalmol 93: 125; 1975

CHAPTER 15

Eyelid reconstruction – anterior lamella

Introduction

The techniques described in this chapter may be used alone to reconstruct the anterior lid lamella in partial thickness defects in which the posterior lamella is intact, or they may be used in combination with techniques described in Chapter 16 to reconstruct both lamellae in full thickness lid defects. When both lid lamellae are reconstructed there must be a blood supply to at least one of them.

Classification: Skin grafts – full thickness
                                            – split thickness
                     Skin flaps – advancement
                                            – rotation
                                            – transposition

Use of flaps to cover defect

Skin flaps used to reconstruct the periocular tissues are almost always local flaps with a random pattern blood supply although distant flaps and those with an axial pattern blood supply are used occasionally. The general rule that random pattern flaps should have a length:breadth ratio of 1:1 can be relaxed in reconstruction of the face because of the rich blood supply compared with the skin of the trunk or limbs. Since skin flaps have an intact blood supply it is not essential for the posterior lamella to be vascularised.

Choice of operation

Guidelines for the use of each flap are given with the description of each procedure.

Advancement flaps

15:2   **Advancement flaps in lower lid**

A simple advancement or sliding flap may be used if the leading edge has to be advanced only a relatively small distance to achieve closure of the defect without undue tension. The flaps may be advanced from the temporal side only or, for a central anterior lamellar defect, from medial and lateral.

15.2a

A basal cell carcinoma of the lid margin has been excised.

15.2b

The posterior lamella has been reconstructed, in this case, with a Hughes' tarso conjunctival flap (see 16.4) anchored laterally with a periosteal flap (arrow) (see 16.5). A full thickness skin graft could be used for the anterior lamella (since the Hughes' flap is vascularised) but in this case a broad skin flap is to be advanced from the temporal side. Alternatively, since a skin flap is being used for the anterior lamella, a graft could have been used for the posterior lamella (see Ch. 16, Sect. A).

Place two skin hooks on the proposed leading edge of the flap and advance the flap over the defect. Undermine the skin widely until the flap lies without tension across the whole defect.

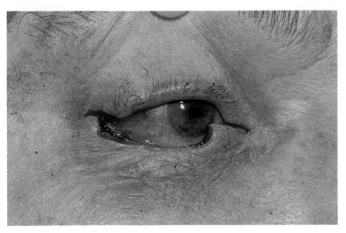

Fig. 15.2a

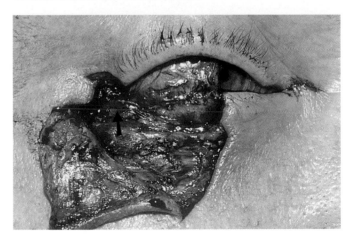

Fig. 15.2b

Technique continues overleaf →

Rotation flaps

A rotation flap is a local flap which can be thought of as several clock-hours of a clock face. The primary defect is created by removing a segment of one or more clock-hours (which includes the lesion) and the remaining clock-hours expand to fill the gap.

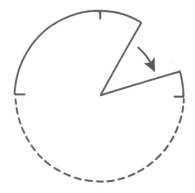

Diag. 15.1

It can be seen that the defect must be triangular with its apex towards the centre of rotation of the flap. A rotation flap does not create a secondary defect which has to be closed. The Mustardé cheek rotation flap is an example.

The Mustardé cheek rotation flap is used to reconstruct large defects of the lower lid up to the whole lid length and, in particular, those defects with a large vertical component. It can also be used for large defects which do not involve the lid margin. By varying the size of the cheek flap smaller defects of the lateral, central or even medial part of the lower lid can be reconstructed with this technique. (See below.)

15:3 **Mustardé cheek rotation flap**

15.3a

Mark the outline of the lesion and the extent of tissue to be excised to remove it. From the medial limit of the tissue to be excised mark a line vertically downwards beside the nose. It should be approximately twice as long as the horizontal extent of the tissue to be excised. From the end of this line draw a second line upwards and laterally to join the lateral limit of the tissue to be excised to create an inverted triangle. From the lateral canthus mark a line which curves upwards towards the lateral end of the eyebrow. If the whole lid is to be reconstructed continue the line in a gentle curve across the temple skin and down just in front of the ear as far as the ear lobe.

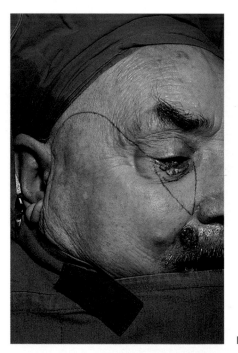

Fig. 15.3a

15.3b

Excise the inverted triangle, including the lesion, staying superficial to the facial muscles unless they are involved with the tumour. Incise the skin to outline the cheek flap. Undermine just deep to the orbicularis muscle as far as the lateral orbital rim. Continue to undermine the cheek flap, dissecting more superficially once the lateral orbital rim has been crossed, within the subcutaneous fat layer, superficial to orbicularis and the facial musculature. The undermining in this plane should continue until the flap can be rotated to fill the defect without undue tension. A back cut at the lower end of the incision by the ear lobe may help to achieve a comfortable rotation of the flap.

15.3c

Reconstruct the posterior lamella using nasal septal cartilage with its mucoperichondrium, or buccal mucous membrane (see 2.13, 2.18). There should be excess mucosa along the superior edge for later reconstruction of the lid margin. If nasal septal cartilage with mucoperichondrium is used, Mustardé recommends that the cartilage should rest on the lower orbital rim to provide support for the lid. Suture the graft to the conjunctiva with interrupted 6/0 absorbable sutures or a 6/0 monofilament suture which can be pulled out.

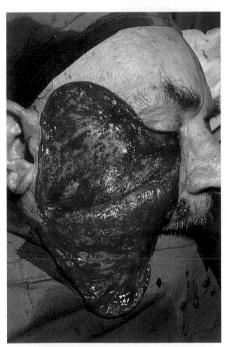

Fig. 15.3b

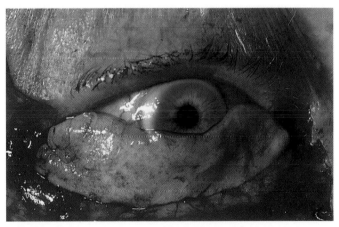

Fig. 15.3c

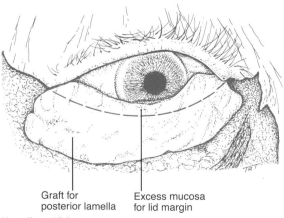

Graft for posterior lamella

Excess mucosa for lid margin

Key diag. 15.3c

Technique continues overleaf ➜

Transposed flaps

A transposed flap is a local flap in which skin is raised on a pedicle at one end and transferred to cover a nearby primary defect. In the face the length : breadth ratio may be greater than 1:1. A secondary defect is created at the donor site which may be closed directly or with a free skin graft.

The design of transposed flaps is important particularly if thicker cheek or forehead skin is to be used. The fundamental point is that the shorter diagonal (AB, Diag.1.2) before the flap is transposed becomes the longer diagonal (BC) after it is transposed (A to C). Allowance must be made, in the design of the flap, for this apparent shortening.

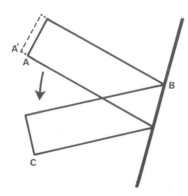

Diag. 15.2

If there is limited elasticity in the flap allowance must also be made for this in designing the flap.

This flap is used for defects in the lower lid which extend to the lateral canthus whether the lid margin is involved (15.5) or not.

15.4a

Mark the skin crease in the upper lid. This will be the inferior border of the flap. Assess the width of flap needed to cover the defect. Draw a line this distance above the marked skin crease. Extend both lines downwards and laterally into healthy skin to the site of the pedicle which should be positioned to allow transposition of the flap to the lid. Assess the length of flap needed, bearing in mind the rules of design outlined above. If in doubt, check that the flap is long enough by placing a length of suture between the superior end of the pedicle laterally and the inferior, medial corner of the defect in the lid. Knot the suture at this point. Now measure from the same point on the pedicle and note where the knot in the suture crosses the skin crease. This is the end of the flap. Tapering of the incision to allow easier closure of the lid, is beyond this point.

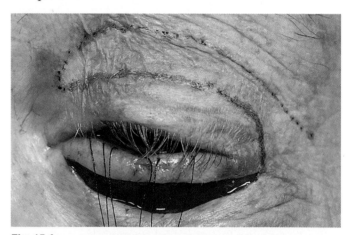

Fig. 15.4a

Upper lid to lower lid transposed flap – lid margin not involved

15.4b

Raise the skin flap. Undermine the skin for a short distance around the pedicle to allow transposition of the flap but take care not to damage the blood supply.

15.4c

Suture the flap into the defect with 6/0 interrupted sutures.

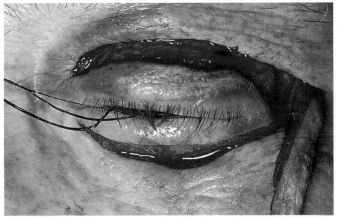

Fig. 15.4b

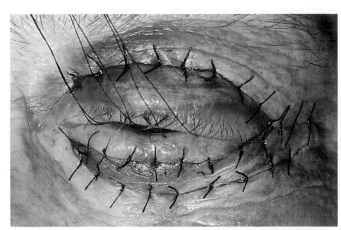

Fig. 15.4c

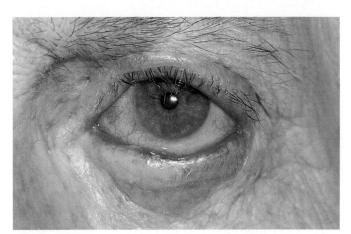

Fig. 15.4 post

15:5 Upper lid to lower lid transposed flap – lid margin involved

15.5a

Assess the width and length of flap required to fill the defect (15.4a)

15.5b

Reconstruct the posterior lamella of the lid with a suitable graft (see Ch. 2, Sect. C; Ch.16, Sect. A) or a tarsoconjunctival flap (see Ch.16, Sect. B). A tarsal graft (see 2.17) was used in the case illustrated. It was supported by a periosteal flap laterally (see 16.5). Raise the skin flap.

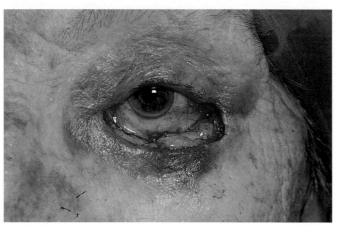

Fig. 15.5a

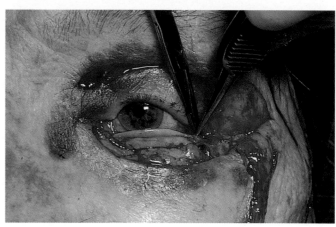

Fig. 15.5b

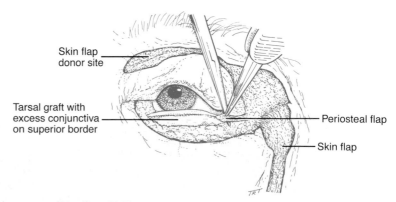

Key diag. 15.5b

Upper lid to lower lid transposed flap – lid margin involved

15.5c

Suture the flap into the defect with a continuous 6/0 monofilament suture along the new lid margin to unite the skin and mucosa (see 15.6e). Use interrupted 6/0 sutures elsewhere. Close the donor site with interrupted 6/0 sutures. Remove all sutures at 5 days.

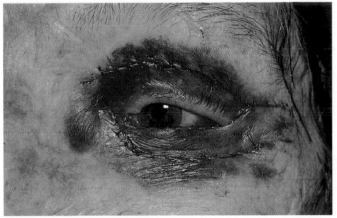

Fig. 15.5c

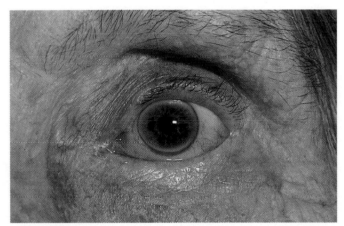

Fig. 15.5 post

Complications and management

Upper lid skin is thin so care must be taken to provide an adequate support in the posterior lamellar reconstruction.

The tip of the flap may show signs of ischaemia in the immediate postoperative period. More survives than seems likely at first.

15:6   Nasojugal transposition flap

15.6a

This flap is used for medial lower lid defects.

15.6b

Reconstruct the posterior lamella with a suitable graft or a tarsoconjunctival flap (see Ch. 16). A tarsal graft was used in the case illustrated. The flap is almost vertical in the nasojugal area with its base just inferior to the medial canthus. Design the flap as described above (see 'Transposed flaps' above; 15.4).

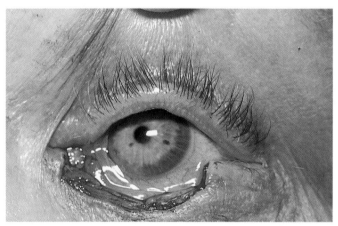

Fig. 15.6a

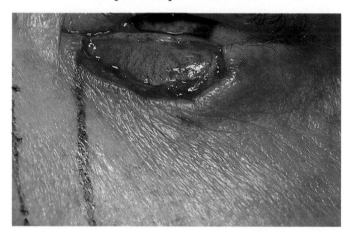

Fig. 15.6b

15.6e

Close the lid margin with a continuous 6/0 suture which unites the skin and the mucosa of the posterior lamellar reconstruction.

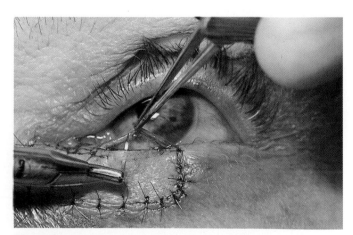

Fig. 15.6e

Nasojugal transposition flap

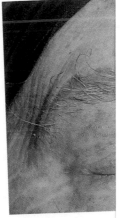

15.7a

Mark an inverted V
forehead. One limb
border of the canth
medial end of the c

Fig. 15.7a

15.7d

Tie the subcutane
excess skin.

15.6c

Raise the flap staying superficial to the facial muscles.

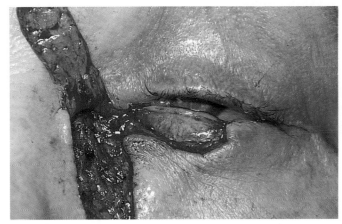

Fig. 15.6c

15.6d

Transpose the flap into the defect. Close the skin with interrupted 6/0 sutures.

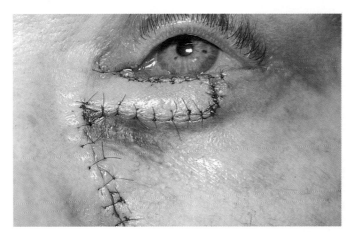

Fig. 15.6d

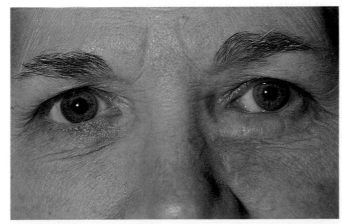

Fig. 15.6 post

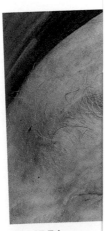

Fig. 15.7d

Complications and management

Nasojugal skin is thicker than eyelid skin and the reconstruction may be rather bulky. Later debulking is possible if necessary.

| 15:7 | **Glabellar V-Y sliding flap** (Continued) |

15.7f

Suture the flap into the canthal defect with 6/0 absorbable sutures to the subcutaneous tissues and 6/0 non-absorbable sutures to the skin. Complete the closure of the forehead. Remove all skin sutures at 1 week.

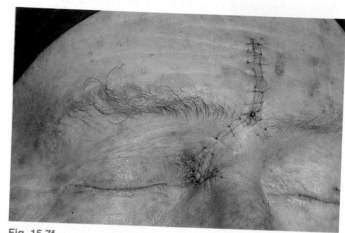

Fig. 15.7f

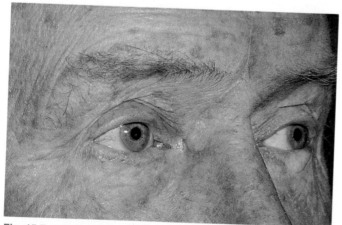

Fig. 15.7 post A and B

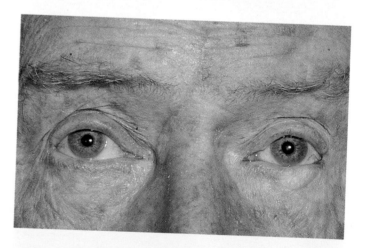

Complications and management

A fold or 'dog-ear' commonly occurs on the bridge of the nose, especially if the defect is large. Leave it for 6 weeks then trim it if necessary. Poor application of the flap to the hollow at the inner canthus, and the appearance of telecanthus, can be avoided by careful placement and suturing of the flap at operation.

15:8 Glabellar transposed flap

15.8a

Mark the defect and estimate whether a glabellar flap alone will be sufficient to reconstruct the lids and canthus.

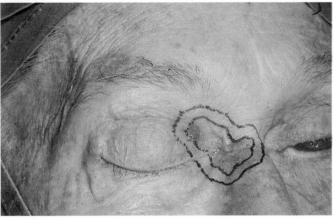

Fig. 15.8a

15.8b

Having excised the tumour, draw the lids medially to estimate the size of flap required. Mark a large glabellar flap extending further up the forehead but otherwise following the principles above (see 15.7a).

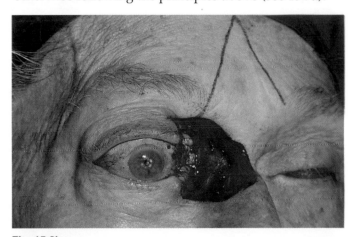

Fig. 15.8b

15.8c

Raise the flap in the subcutaneous fat layer and undermine the forehead skin at either side to minimise tension across the wound when the forehead is closed.

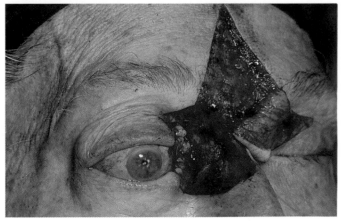

Fig. 15.8c

Technique continues overleaf →

Grafts to reconstruct the posterior lamella

Choice of operation

In the upper lid oral mucous membrane, tarsal plate from the opposite upper lid, or a tarsomarginal graft are used.

In the lower lid the posterior lamella must provide added support because of the effect of gravity. Oral mucosa alone will not be sufficient to support a thin skin flap; it may be acceptable, although not ideal, as a lining for a thicker flap. In general a graft of sclera, tarsal plate or cartilage is preferable.

Preparing the grafts

See Chapter 2, Section D, for methods of taking oral mucous membrane, auricular cartilage, tarsal plate and sclera. See 16.2 for the method of taking nasal septal cartilage with mucoperichondrium.

16:1   Use of grafts for the posterior lamella

The posterior lamellar graft must be sutured to tarsal plate or canthal tendon, at the ends of the defect, with interrupted or continuous 6/0 catgut or a longer acting absorbable suture (see 15.3c, 15.5b, 15.6b,c). If the canthal tissues are absent medially the attachment should be to the periosteum posterior to the normal attachment of the medial canthal tendon with two 4/0 or 5/0 non-absorbable sutures. Laterally, a new canthal tendon may be reconstructed with a flap of periosteum (see 16.5).

Suture together the free edges of the skin and the posterior lamellar graft, at the lid margin, with a continuous 6/0 monofilament suture. If mucosa has been used for the posterior lamella there should be a sufficient excess to extend over the lid margin and allow suture to the skin (see 15.3d). Similarly, a tarsal graft should have excess conjunctiva at its superior border (see 15.5b, 15.6e).

Complications and management

Some degree of contraction occurs with all posterior lamellar grafts. Those without a mucosal lining may cause irritation until they are epithelialised.

Alternative procedures

16:2   Nasal septal cartilage with mucoperichondrium

This cartilage graft has the advantage over auricular cartilage (see 2.16) of being lined with mucosa although it is rather thick mucosa. The cartilage, also, is thicker than auricular cartilage but it provides a useful support in some situations such as a Mustardé cheek rotation flap (see 15.3).

Bleeding may be reduced by packing the nose in the anaesthetic room with ribbon gauze soaked in 4% cocaine. In theatre inject 1:200 000 adrenaline submucosally on one side of the septum. Insert a nasal speculum on the side opposite to the injection. Adequate access to the nasal septum can usually be obtained with a nasal speculum alone. If difficulty is experienced the exposure is improved by incising through the alar base and elevating the lateral wall of the nostril.

Incise the nasal septal mucosa just above and parallel to the mucocutaneous junction within the nose. Deepen the incision to make a partial thickness cut through the septal cartilage.

Cut through the remaining cartilage with a Rollett's rougine. Take care not to perforate the opposite perichondrium and mucosa. If a perforation is made suture it with 6/0 plain catgut.

Dissect the intact mucoperichondrium from the opposite side of the cartilage using a blunt periosteal elevator, e.g. MacDonald.

Protect the intact mucoperichondrium with the blunt dissector and cut the graft of cartilage and attached mucosa with scissors from each end of the original incision.

Use angled scissors or a blade to cut the proximal end of the composite graft. Shave to reduce the cartilage, if necessary, to the required thickness.

Repair the alar base if it was opened.

To dress the nose cut two fingers from an operating glove, pack each with paraffin gauze and lubricate each with liquid paraffin. Place one finger in each side of the nose. Remove on the first postoperative day and use antibiotic and vasoconstrictive drops for a month.

> **Complications and management**
>
> If the intact mucosa of the opposite side of the nose is incised close the defect with interrupted 6/0 catgut sutures.

16:3   Tarsomarginal graft

Since a defect of a quarter of the length of an eyelid margin can be closed direct free grafts of this size, which include the lid margin, may be excised from one or more of the normal lids and used to reconstruct an upper or lower lid defect. The skin and orbicularis muscle are removed from the surface of the graft but the lid margin and lashes are left intact. The graft of tarsal plate and lid margin is sutured into the defect and covered with a local skin flap. There should be minimal tension across the graft(s) when sutured into the defect. Remove all skin sutures at 5 days and the lid margin sutures at 7 days.

Since the blood supply is from the skin flap two or even three tarsomarginal grafts may be sutured in a row to reconstruct larger defects.

> **Complications and management**
>
> The graft may necrose particularly if there is any tension across it. The resulting notch may be excised when healing has occurred, after 3–6 months, and the defect reconstructed by an alternative method.

Flaps to reconstruct the posterior lamella

Choice of operation

The only posterior lamellar flap is tarsal plate with its blood supply intact through a pedicle of conjunctiva. Tarsus is always taken from the upper lid to reconstruct the lower lid and not vice versa because the lower tarsal plate is too narrow to use in the upper lid. The Hughes' tarsoconjunctival flap (16.4) is the most commonly used but variations have been described, including the use of a local tarsoconjunctival flap to reconstruct an adjacent area in the ipsilateral upper lid.

The lateral canthal tendon may be reconstructed to support the lateral canthus by fashioning a flap of periosteum (16.5) at the lateral orbital rim. Support at the medial canthus relies on direct attachment to the periosteum or to a transnasal wire (see 18.3)

16:4 Hughes' tarsoconjunctival flap

A broad strip of upper tarsal plate on a pedicle of conjunctiva is used to reconstruct the posterior lamella of the lower lid. It may be covered with a skin graft (16.4g) or flap (see 15.2b,c). The pedicle is divided after a few weeks.

16.4a

The use of the Hughes' flap is restricted to relatively shallow lower lid defects which do not extend much beyond the inferior border of the tarsal plate.

16.4b

Estimate the length of posterior lamella required (see 'Introduction').

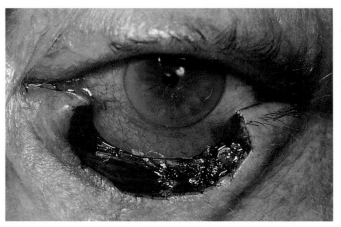

Fig. 16.4a

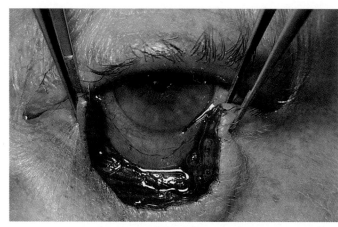

Fig. 16.4b

16.4e

Identify Muller's muscle as it inserts along the superior tarsal border and carefully dissect it free taking care not to damage the underlying conjunctiva. This reduces the risk of upper lid retraction following the second stage of the procedure. There will be moderate haemorrhage from the large vessels on the surface of Muller's muscle but be careful not to cauterise the conjunctival vessels. Continue the dissection between Muller's muscle and the conjunctiva for about 10mm superiorly. Allow Muller's muscle to retract where it has been freed. Extend the vertical tarsal cuts for 3–4mm into the conjunctiva to lengthen the tarsoconjunctival flap.

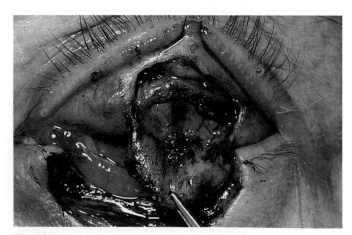

Fig. 16.4e

16.4c

Evert the upper lid and measure 4 mm from the lid margin.

16.4d

Insert a stay suture of 4/0 silk through the tarsal plate close to the lid margin and evert the lid over a Desmarres retractor. Mark a line 4 mm from and parallel to the lid margin. Mark on this line the horizontal length of tarsal plate required. From these marks draw vertical lines (arrows) to the superior tarsal border to delineate the flap. Incise the tarsal plate through its full thickness along the marks to enter the easily identified pretarsal space. Raise the U-shaped flap of tarsus by dissection in the pretarsal space as far as the superior border of the tarsal plate.

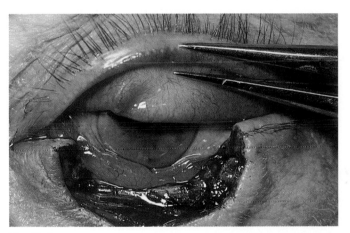

Fig. 16.4c

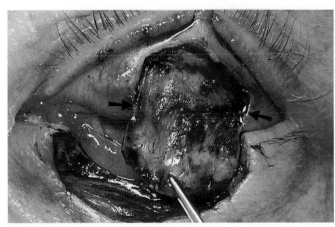

Fig. 16.4d

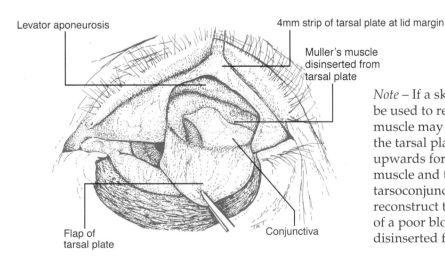

Levator aponeurosis

4mm strip of tarsal plate at lid margin

Muller's muscle disinserted from tarsal plate

Flap of tarsal plate

Conjunctiva

Note – If a skin graft, especially if it is rather thick, is to be used to reconstruct the anterior lamella, Muller's muscle may be left attached to the superior border of the tarsal plate to improve the blood supply. Dissect upwards for a few millimetres between Muller's muscle and the levator aponeurosis to mobilise the tarsoconjunctival flap. If a skin flap is to be used to reconstruct the anterior lamella there will be little risk of a poor blood supply and Muller's muscle should be disinserted from the tarsus as described above.

Key diag. 16.4e

Technique continues overleaf →

16:4 **Hughes' tarsoconjunctival flap** *(Continued)*

16.4f

Suture the flap into the defect with 6/0 catgut sutures. Begin by suturing the ends of the superior border of the upper tarsal plate to the lower lid margins at the edges of the defect. Suture the remaining edges of the tarsus to the conjunctiva.

16.4g

Reconstruct the anterior lamella with a full thickness skin graft (see 2.7, 2.8) or a local flap of skin and muscle (see 15.2b, c). In this case skin from the upper lid was used. The anterior lamellar reconstruction must be slightly convex superiorly to cover the tarsal plate without tension. This will flatten when the pedicle is divided.

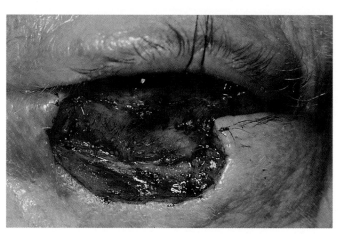

Fig. 16.4f

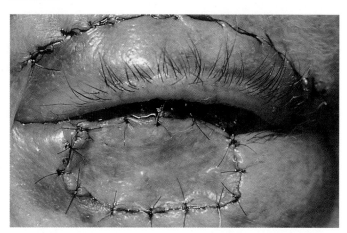

Fig. 16.4g

16.4h

After about 3 weeks divide the pedicle 2–3 mm superior to the tarsal plate and skin graft. Suture the free edge of the conjunctiva to the skin with a continuous 6/0 monofilament suture. Remove this suture at 5 days.

The upper lid retractors will have been advanced by the procedure and must be recessed to prevent upper lid retraction. To do this dissect between the conjunctiva and the retractors until the lid is at a satisfactory level. Allow the proximal conjunctiva to retract. A downward traction suture on the upper lid for 24 hours may be needed.

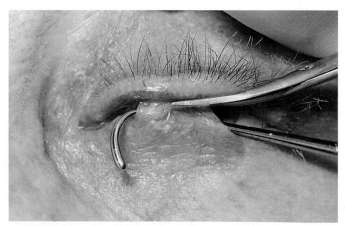

Fig. 16.4h

Hughes' tarsoconjunctival flap

16.5a

This technique is used to support the upper or lower lid, or both, laterally when the lateral canthal tendon is inadequate. It is useful in lid reconstruction when lateral fixation of the posterior lamella is required (see 15.2b, 15.5b), or in any situation where the tendon is lax or absent and the lateral canthus has moved medially (the case illustrated).

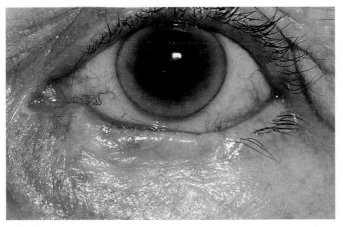

Fig. 16.4 post

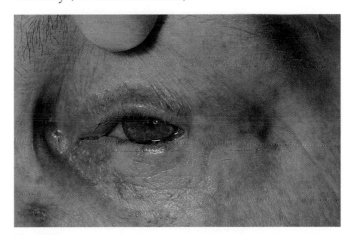

Fig. 16.5a

Complications and management

Retraction of the upper lid may follow the second stage if the upper lid tissues have not been freed sufficiently. Dissect further between the conjunctiva and the upper lid retractors until the lid is at the correct level.

Technique continues overleaf →

16:5 **Lateral periosteal flap** *(Continued)*

16.5b

Make a horizontal incision from the lateral canthus to expose the lateral orbital rim. At the level of the lateral canthal tendon mark two horizontal lines on the periosteum, 8–10 mm apart, extending from the medial border of the lateral orbital rim to the temporalis fascia laterally. If support for both lids is required cut a broader strip of periosteum to allow it to be split later. Mark the lateral extent of the flap with a vertical line.

16.5c

Incise the edges of the flap leaving the periosteum intact medially and lift the flap of periosteum with a periosteal elevator. Leave the base of the flap attached to the periosteum within the lateral rim of the orbit.

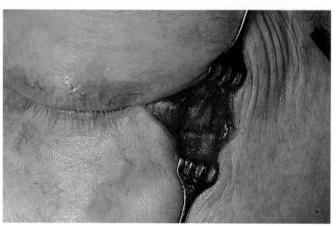

Fig. 16.5b

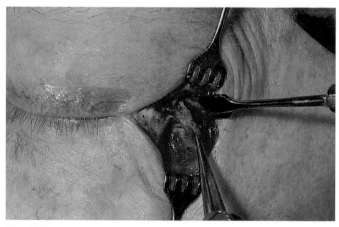

Fig. 16.5c

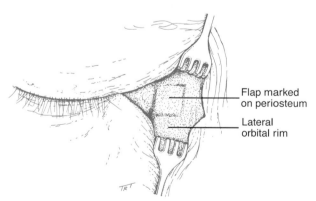

Flap marked on periosteum

Lateral orbital rim

Key diag. 16.5b

16.5d

To attach the canthal tissues or the reconstructed posterior lamella to the periosteal flap pass one or two double-armed 5/0 non-absorbable sutures through the lid tissues then pass both needles through the periosteal flap.

16.5e

Tie the sutures to support the lid tissues. There should be minimal horizontal lid laxity. If a broader strip of periosteum has been cut for the support of both lids split it into an upper and a lower limb and attach them to the posterior lamellae of the upper and lower lids in the same way.

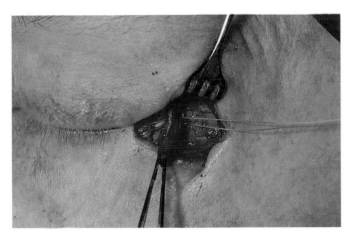

Fig. 16.5d

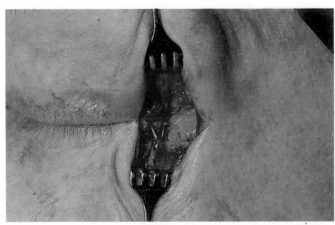

Fig. 16.5e

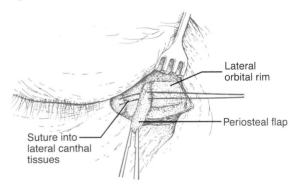

Lateral orbital rim

Periosteal flap

Suture into lateral canthal tissues

Key diag. 16.5d

Technique continues overleaf →

| 16:5 | Lateral periosteal flap |

FURTHER READING

Mehotra O N: Repairing defects of the lower eyelid with a free chondromucosal graft. Plast Reconstr Surg 59: 689; 1977

Putterman A M: Combined viable composite graft and temporal semicircular skin flap procedure. Am J Ophthalmol 98: 349; 1984

Siegel R J: Palatal grafts for eyelid reconstruction. Ophthalm Plast Reconstr Surg 76: 411; 1985

Stephenson C M, Brown B Z: The use of tarsus as a free autogenous graft in eyelid surgery. Ophthalm Plast Reconstr Surg 1: 43, 1985

| 16.5f |

Close the incision in two layers.

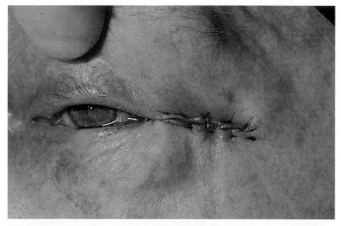

Fig. 16.5f

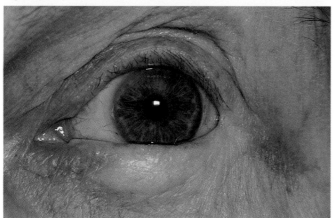

Fig. 16.5 post

Complications and management

Care is needed in the design of the flap to ensure that the canthus is held at the correct level. With time some relaxation of the flap may occur.

CHAPTER 17

Eyelid reconstruction – anterior and posterior lamellae combined

An alternative to the separate reconstruction of each lamella of an eyelid is to use a flap which combines both lamellae. Full thickness eyelid flaps are used. Since a normally functioning upper lid should be protected these flaps are taken only from the lower lid for reconstruction of the upper lid.

Choice of operation

The two techniques described are used for defects of more than one-third length. The more commonly used is the Cutler-Beard bridge flap (17.1). The 'switch flap' (17.2), which is less commonly used, can provide an excellent reconstruction of large upper lid defects with the preservation of most of the lashes but a subsequent reconstruction of the lower lid, including the margin, is required. The disadvantage of both techniques, when compared with techniques which do not require a bridge between the lids, is that the eye is closed for several weeks between the two stages.

17:1 Cutler–Beard flap

This is a two-stage technique for reconstruction of large full thickness defects in the upper lid. It may be combined with a glabellar flap for large medial defects (see 15.9).

17.1a

Having created the defect pull gently on the edges to estimate the residual defect which has to be reconstructed. This is the horizontal width of the bridge flap. Draw a horizontal line 5mm inferior and parallel to the lash line of the lower lid. Mark the width of flap required on this line and draw two vertical lines as far as the inferior orbital rim.

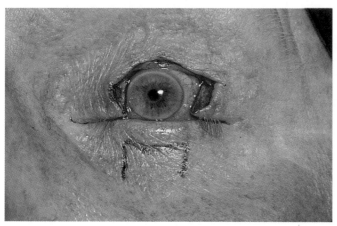

Fig. 17.1a

17.1b

Incise along the lines. Perforate the full thickness of the lid at the corners of the flap and with a pair of scissors inserted between the stab incisions complete the horizontal full thickness incision. Extend this inferiorly along the vertical lines to the inferior conjunctival fornix to create a U-shaped flap. Pull the flap up posterior to the lower lid margin.

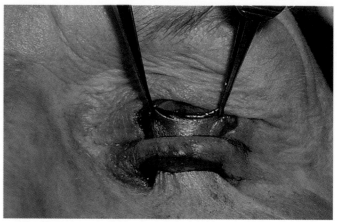

Fig. 17.1b

17.1e

Suture the conjunctiva to skin, over the new lid margin, with a 6/0 continuous monofilament suture. Remove this at 5 days. Replace the pedicle of the bridge into the lower lid defect and repair it in layers to avoid a fistula through the lid.

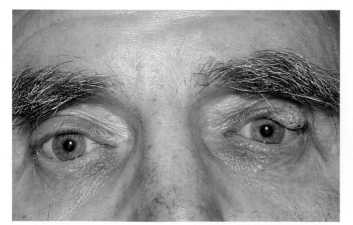

Fig. 17.1 pre

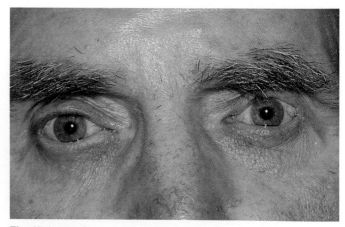

Fig. 17.1 post A

17.1c

Suture it into the upper lid defect in three layers: conjunctiva to conjunctiva, and orbicularis muscle of the lower lid to the levator aponeurosis and orbicularis muscle of the upper lid, with interrupted 6/0 absorbable sutures. Finally, skin to skin with 6/0 interrupted non-absorbable sutures. Remove the sutures at 5 days.

17.1d

After 6 weeks estimate whether the flap has stretched enough to reduce the tension. If it is still tight leave it another 3–6 weeks. If it has strectched and feels less tight divide the bridge to restore the upper lid margin. To do this pass a squint hook posterior to the flap and carefully incise the layers of the flap making the initial incision convex downwards to allow for retraction. Leave an excess of conjunctiva.

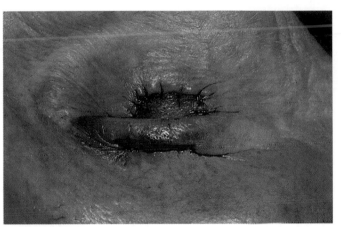

Fig. 17.1c

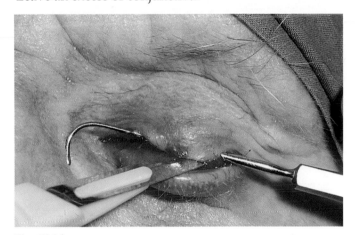

Fig. 17.1d

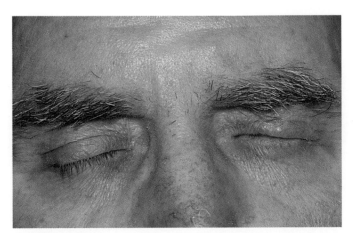

Fig. 17.1 post B

Complications and management

Necrosis of the lower lid margin may occur if the marginal artery was damaged when the flap was cut. Wait until the second stage of the procedure and attempt to close the surviving marginal tissues, with a cantholysis or other procedure if necessary.

The reconstructed upper lid margin is relatively unstable and may become entropic. The margin may be irregular at the edges of the bridge flap. Allow the lid to heal and excise the notches if necessary. Skin hairs may cause irritation and they can be treated with cryotherapy as described in Chapter 8.

Alternative procedure

17:2 **'Switch' flap to the upper lid**

This technique transfers full thickness lower lid, together with the lashes, into the upper lid defect. The lashes are shorter than natural upper lid lashes but they may be preferable to no lashes at all at the site of the reconstruction. The technique is in two stages. At the second stage the pedicle is divided and the lower lid is reconstructed.

Having created the defect in the upper lid gently pull the edges inwards to estimate its true size. Mark the lower lid flap equal in size horizontally and vertically to this (reduced) defect. Leave at least 2 mm between the flap and the lacrimal punctu.

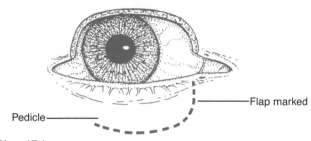

Pedicle ——————

—————— Flap marked

Diag. 17.1

The siting of the pedicle of the flap can influence the final cosmetic result. The principle is that the suture line which is created between the 'switch' flap and the upper lid at the first stage of the procedure may show less scarring than the suture line created by closing the upper lid at the second stage. The junction of the switch flap and the upper lid, created at the first operation, should therefore be the suture line closest to the centre of the upper lid. To achieve this the following rule applies: the pedicle is sited at the lateral end of the flap unless there is a large medial remnant in the upper lid in which case it is sited medially.

Having decided on the site of the pedicle Mustardé recommends that its width should be 5 mm in flaps up to half lid width and 7 mm if more than one-half. Cut the flap starting at the end opposite to the pedicle, taking care not to damage the vascular supply in the pedicle.

If the lower lid defect created by rotating the flap is less than one-quarter of lid length it will be possible to close the lower lid directly. Close it as far as possible at this stage without disturbing the circulation in the pedicle. If the defect is more than one-quarter of lid length the lower lid reconstruction will all be at the second stage.

Suture the flap into the upper lid defect as far as possible, using the standard technique and taking care of the pedicle.

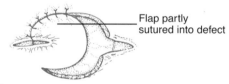

—————— Flap partly
sutured into defect

Diag. 17.2

Two to three weeks later divide the pedicle. Freshen the exposed edges to allow accurate closure of the pedicle end of the flap to the upper lid. Close the upper lid in layers as usual.

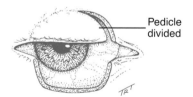

—————— Pedicle
divided

Diag. 17.3

'Switch' flap to the upper lid

FURTHER READING

Cutler N L, Beard C: A method for partial and total upper lid reconstruction. Am J Ophthalmol 39: 1; 1955

Mustardé J C: Repair and reconstruction in the orbital region, 3rd edn. Churchill Livingstone, Edinburgh; 1991

Closure of the lower lid defect

If direct closure was planned freshen the edges of the exposed tissues and complete the closure started at the first stage. If direct closure was not planned reconstruct the lower lid with any appropriate technique as discussed in Chapters 14–16. The choice is limited because no upper lid tissues are available. However, skin is usually available laterally. A lateral cantholysis (see 14.1) may be all that is required for smaller defects. Larger defects may require a semicircular flap (see 14.2) or a cheek rotation flap of appropriate size (see 14.3, 15.3).

Complications and management

Damage to the vascular supply in the pedicle will cause ischaemia in the flap. If this occurs while cutting the flap return the flap to the lower lid and wait for a week before rotating the flap into the upper lid. Later ischaemia may not result in total loss of the flap. Divide the pedicle at the normal time.

Oedema of the reconstructed upper lid is common but it usually settles within a few weeks.

Contracture in either suture line in the upper lid may result in a notch. Wait 6 months then excise the notch (see 2.6).

Epicanthus and/or telecanthus

Choice of operation

Correct large epicanthic folds with a Mustardé double Z-plasty (18.1). Smaller folds may be corrected with the simpler Y–V plasty (18.2). In telecanthus the medial canthal tendon after shortening must be refixed to the side of the nose in the region of the anterior or posterior lacrimal crest. If the bony anatomy is normal fix it to the periosteum just posterior to the original tendon insertion (18.1e) or to the posterior lacrimal crest periosteum. If surgery to the bones is needed to correct a congenital deformity or the effects of trauma, fix the tendon with a transnasal wire (18.3).

18:1 Mustardé double Z-plasty

This technique may be used to correct epicanthic folds and/or telecanthus. In telecanthus the eyes (and orbits) are in a normal position but the intercanthal distance is greater than half the interpupillary distance. The correction of epicanthic folds with telecanthus is illustrated but the technique may be used for either alone. In any midfacial congenital abnormality look for and correct any underlying bony craniofacial anomaly before surgery to the soft tissues.

18.1a

Mark the site of the intended medial canthus (A) on each side. The distance between the marks should be half the interpupillary distance. If there is no telecanthus each mark will lie directly over the existing canthus but on the anterior face of the epicanthic fold. If telecanthus is present each mark will lie medial to the existing canthus.

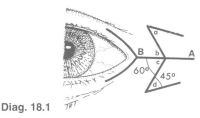

Diag. 18.1

Pull the skin towards the midline to obliterate each epicanthic fold in turn and mark the site of the existing canthus (B). Join the two marks, A and B (see Diag. 18.1). Bisect the line and draw two further lines, 2 mm shorter than A–B and at 60 degrees to A–B. From their ends draw lines of the same length at 45 degrees. Finally draw two lines of the same length from B close to the upper and lower lid margins.

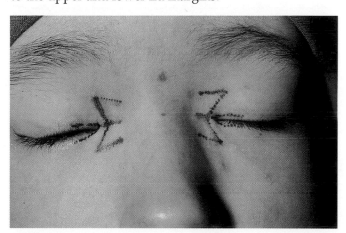

Fig. 18.1a

18.1b

Incise the skin along the lines.

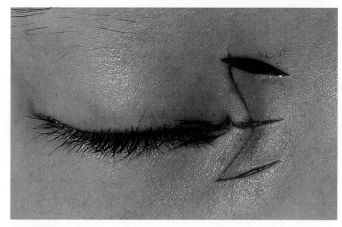

Fig. 18.1b

Technique continues overleaf ➔

18:1   **Mustardé double Z-plasty** *(Continued)*

18.1c

Undermine the flaps and retract them with stay sutures.

18.1d

Carefully excise the exposed subcutaneous tissue, which includes orbicularis muscle and the fat deep to it, to expose the medial canthal tendon. The periosteum on the side of the nose will be exposed medially. The angular vein will be encountered and should be preserved if possible.

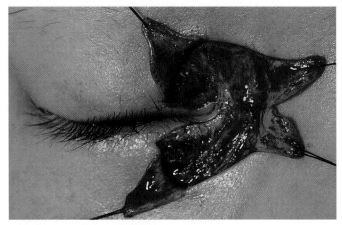

Fig. 18.1c

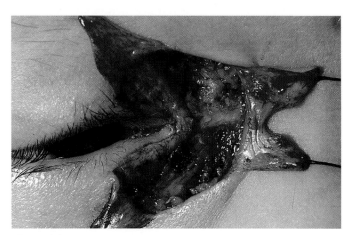

Fig. 18.1d

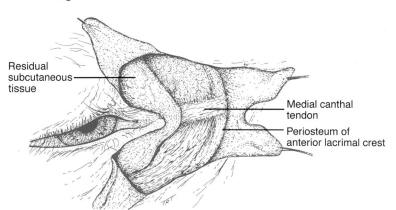

Key diag. 18.1d

Residual subcutaneous tissue

Medial canthal tendon

Periosteum of anterior lacrimal crest

Mustardé double Z-plasty

18.1e

To correct telecanthus, if present, cut the medial canthal tendon taking care not to damage the underlying lacrimal apparatus. Pass both ends of a double-armed 4/0 non-absorbable suture from posterior to anterior through the lateral part of the tendon close to the medial canthus. Pass the needles through the original insertion of the medial canthal tendon. Begin just posterior to the insertion and pass the needles forward through the periosteum and the insertion and tie them anteriorly. This ensures that the medial canthus is not pulled anteriorly.

18.1f

Tie the suture (arrow) to draw the canthal tissue medially.

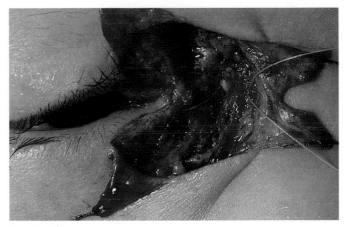

Fig. 18.1e

Fig. 18.1f

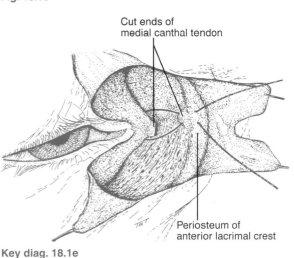

Cut ends of
medial canthal tendon

Periosteum of
anterior lacrimal crest

Key diag. 18.1e

As an alternative a transnasal wire (18.3) may be used to fix the canthi.

If no telecanthus is present the medial canthal tendon is not disturbed.

Technique continues overleaf ➔

18:1 **Mustardé double Z-plasty** *(Continued)*

18.1g

18.1g Transpose the flaps a and b and c and d (see Diag. 18.1). It may be necessary to trim the flaps to achieve a comfortable fit but be careful not to trim too much. Close the skin with 6/0 catgut. A 6/0 non-absorbable suture may be used in an adult and removed after 5 days.

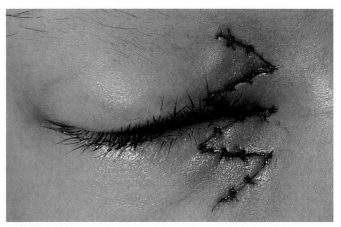

Fig. 18.1g

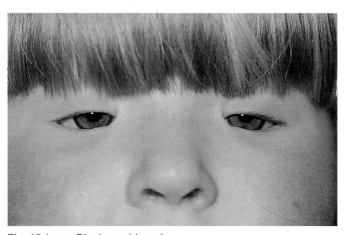

Fig. 18.1 pre Blepharophimosis

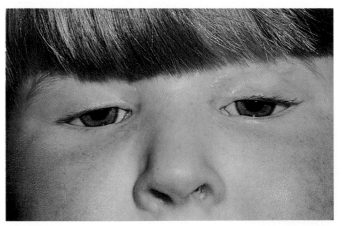

Fig. 18.1 post Ptosis to be corrected

Complications and management

The scars are usually rather obvious for several months but in time they soften and blend well into the surrounding skin.

Undercorrection of the telecanthus or late drift of the canthi laterally may be corrected with a transnasal wire (18.3) if not used primarily.

Alternative procedure

18:2 Y–V plasty

If the epicanthic folds are small this technique may be used instead of a double Z-plasty.

Mark the intended site of the new medial canthus (A) and the existing medial canthus (B). Join the marks. From B draw lines equal in length to A–B close to the upper and lower lid margins.

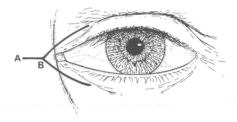

Diag. 18.2

Incise the lines and remove subcutaneous tissue (see 18.1d) to expose the medial canthal tendon. Shorten the tendon as above. Close the Y-shaped incision as a V. If the new medial canthus is found to be significantly posterior to the point A it may be necessary to close the incision as a Y.

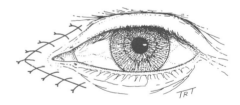

Diag. 18.3

18:3　Transnasal wire to fix the canthi

If the anterior lacrimal crests are prominent or displaced laterally to any degree the refixation of the shortened medial canthal tendons will be unsatisfactory and the telecanthus will probably be undercorrected. A transnasal wire will result in a better correction.

In traumatic telecanthus, especially if there have been fractures in the region of the lacrimal fossa, a transnasal wire is preferred to direct refixation of the medial canthal tendon to the periosteum. A double Z-plasty, Y–V incision or oblique straight incision may be used. If the canthus is displaced superiorly or inferiorly a Z-plasty (see 18.4) allows the vertical displacement to be corrected before a transnasal wire is inserted.

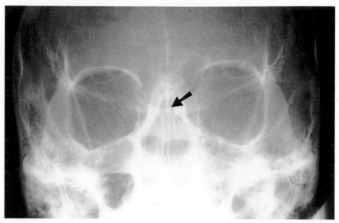

Fig. 18.3 XR1 Cribriform plate in the normal position

In unilateral cases the transnasal wire is anchored around the medial canthal tendon on the normal side and acts as an anchor for the medial canthal tissues on the affected side. In bilateral cases the transnasal wire anchors the medial canthal tissues on both sides which pull against each other across the nose.

Before operation it is important to establish that the cribriform plate (arrow) is in a normal position. If it is low the wire would enter the anterior cranial fossa and cause a leak of cerebrospinal fluid – an alternative method of fixation should be used.

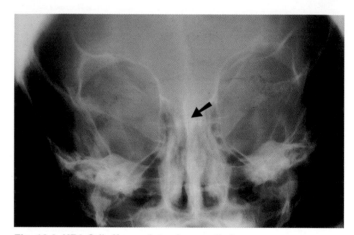

Fig. 18.3 XR2 Cribriform plate abnormally low

18.3a

In unilateral cases mark and incise the skin and remove the subcutaneous tissue to expose the medial canthal tendon (see 18.1a–d). In traumatic cases the tendon may have been destroyed. In the case illustrated a left unilateral telecanthus is being corrected. A left dacryocystorhinostomy was performed at the same time and bilateral straight incisions have been used.

18.3b

In unilateral cases incise the periosteum of the anterior lacrimal crest, strip the periosteum laterally together with the medial canthal tendon and lacrimal sac until the lacrimal fossa is clearly exposed. Make a large osteum, 10–15 mm diameter, in the floor of the lacrimal fossa and excise part of the anterior lacrimal crest as for a dacryocystorhinostomy. Note that a dacryocystorhinostomy can be performed at this stage in the procedure if indicated.

On the opposite side expose the medial canthal tendon through a dacryocystorhinostomy incision and do not cut it. Incise the periosteum of the anterior lacrimal crest inferior to the medial canthal tendon and reflect it laterally with the lacrimal sac to expose the lacrimal fossa, leaving the medial canthal tendon intact. Place a stay suture around it.

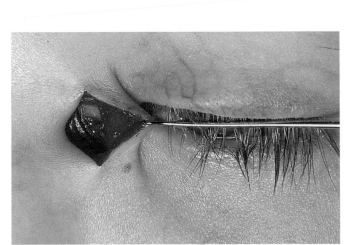

Fig. 18.3a

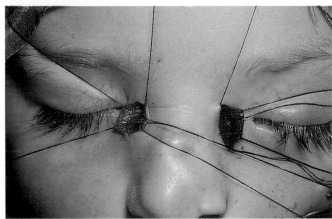

Fig. 18.3b

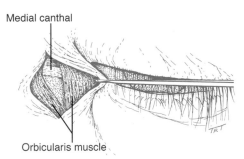

Key diag. 18.3a

In bilateral cases cut the medial canthal tendon, reflect the lacrimal sac, make a large osteum in the floor of the lacrimal fossa and trim the anterior lacrimal crest on both sides.

In bilateral cases repeat the procedure on the opposite side.

Technique continues overleaf ➔

18.3c

Take a 15 cm length of stainless steel wire (36 gauge, 0.16 mm diameter is suitable) and a length of 4/0 monofilament nylon and introduce them into the eye of an awl such as a Mustardé awl. Place an artery clip on one end of each.

18.3d

In unilateral cases place a metal guard to protect the eye on the affected side. Pass the awl from the normal side through the osteum in the floor of the lacrimal fossa as far posteriorly as possible.

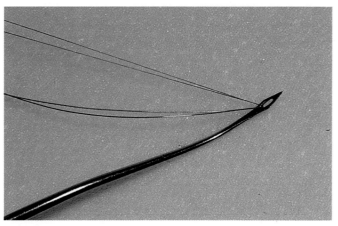

Fig. 18.3c

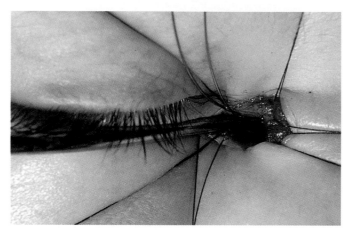

Fig. 18.3d

In bilateral cases the wire can be introduced from either side.

18.3g

In unilateral cases, having withdrawn the awl back across the nose and removed it, pass one end of the wire beneath the medial canthal tendon on the normal side so that one end of the wire lies each side of the tendon.

In bilateral cases place the tip of an artery forceps between the two limbs of the wire, close to the osteum in the lacrimal fossa ready for the wires to be wound around it.

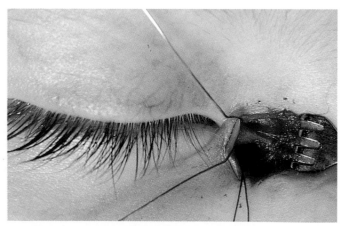

Fig. 18.3g

18.3e

Direct the awl across the posterior part of the nose to exit in the floor of the lacrimal fossa against the guard (arrow) protecting the eye.

18.3f

Pull through the unclipped end of the nylon suture and clip it. This suture now lies freely through the nose with a clip on each end. Introduce a new length of nylon suture into the eye of the awl and clip one end.

Holding the looped end of the wire firmly in artery forceps, carefully withdraw the awl back across the nose. Leave a clip on the loop of wire.

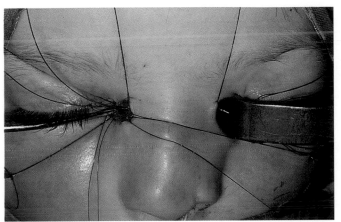

Fig. 18.3e

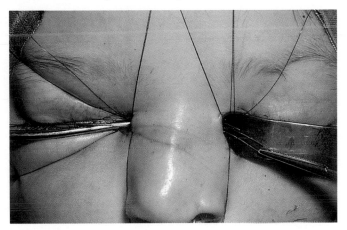

Fig. 18.3f

Pull through the unclipped end of the second nylon suture and clip it. It now lies feely through the nose with a clip on each end. Remove the awl from the free end of the wire.

18.3h

In unilateral cases wind the ends of the wire together over the medial canthal tendon on the normal side.

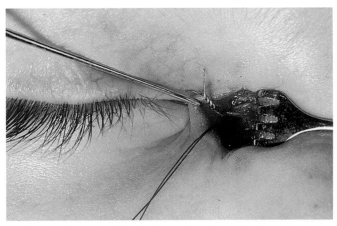

In bilateral cases wind the free ends of the wire together over the tip of the artery clip to create a loop. Do not tighten the wire at this stage.

Fig. 18.3h

Technique continues overleaf ➜

18:3   **Transnasal wire to fix the canthi** *(Continued)*

18.3i

In unilateral cases place a probe in the lower canaliculus. Pass one or two 4/0 monofilament nylon or braided stainless steel wire sutures through the tissues of the medial canthus then through the loop in the transnasal wire (arrows). Tie these sutures.

18.3j

Now twist the wire ends more tightly until a satisfactory correction of the telecanthus is achieved. During this manoeuvre the medial canthal tendon or the canthal suture must be held free of the turns in the wire. Trim the ends of the wire and turn the ends to face medially.

Using a curved needle with an eye pass the ends of the nylon sutures through the skin of the posterior wound edge, close to the inner canthi. Close the skin incisions with interrupted 6/0 sutures.

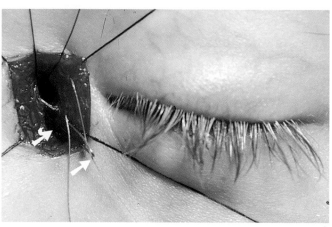

Fig. 18.3i

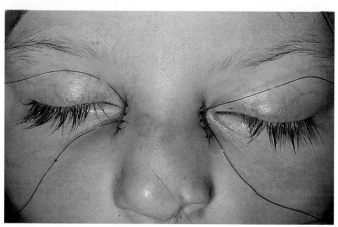

Fig. 18.3j

In bilateral cases repeat on the opposite side.

18.3k

Tie the nylon sutures over a bolster on each side to maintain the shape of the new canthi.

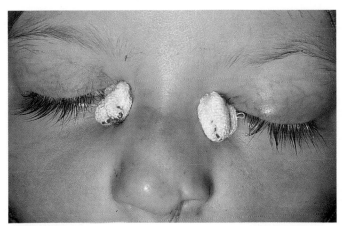

Fig. 18.3k

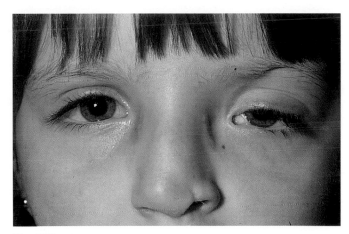

Fig. 18.3 pre

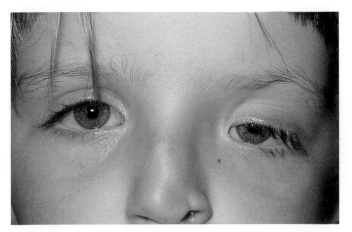

Fig. 18.3 post Ptosis to be corrected.

Remove the bolsters and skin sutures after 5 days.

Complications and management

The position of the canthi may be too anterior if the wire is not passed well posteriorly through the nose. Some lateral drift of the canthi may occur with time.

Vertical displacement of the medial canthus

18:4 Z-plasty to medial canthus

This technique may be combined with a Lester Jones tube if the lacrimal apparatus has been destroyed. However, it is usually safer to allow the canthus to heal fully first.

The case illustrated has bilateral traumatic anophthalmos with multiple middle third facial fractures which have been reduced as far as possible.

18.4a

Mark the existing canthus and the intended site of the new canthus. Mark a Z based on these positions. Attempt to probe the lacrimal canaliculi and syringe the lacrimal drainage system to assess its patency.

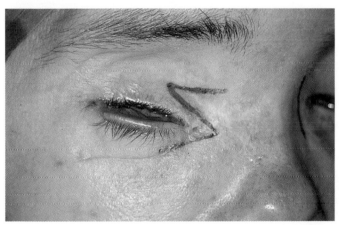

Fig. 18.4a

18.4b

Incise the Z and the underlying tissue. Undermine to allow comfortable transposition of the flaps. If the lacrimal drainage system is intact place probes in the canaliculi during this dissection.

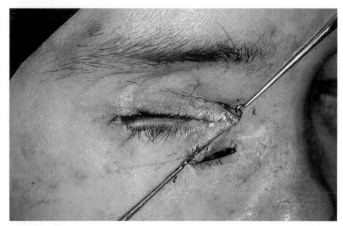

Fig. 18.4b

Technique continues overleaf ➜

18:4 | **Z-plasty to medial canthus** *(Continued)*

18.4c

Secure the canthus in its new position with a transnasal wire as described above.

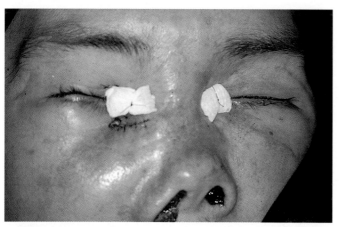

Fig. 18.4c

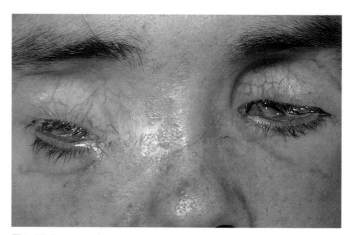

Fig. 18.4 pre

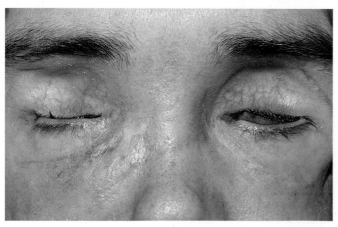

Fig. 18.4 post

Complications and management

Distortion of the canthus may occur if the flaps cannot be transposed easily. If the lacrimal drainage apparatus is intact its function may be compromised.

Orbital decompression

Orbital decompression is indicated most commonly in sight-threatening thyroid eye disease. This includes deteriorating visual acuity, visual field or colour vision (as a result of optic nerve compression) which does not respond to high steroid dosage (70–100 mg prednisolone daily) or which recurs after the steroid treatment is reduced. Other indications are the inability to take steroids for any reason and exposure of the cornea which, because of the degree of proptosis, cannot be fully corrected by lid surgery alone.

The preoperative assessment must include the parameters under threat listed above plus the pupil reactions, intraocular pressures, eye movements and degree of proptosis. The margin-reflex distance to all four lids should also be noted (see 3.1)

Bilateral decompressions at the same operation may be needed. Probably the most satisfactory decompression follows removal of the medial wall and floor of the orbit. The most familiar approach for the ophthalmologist is through a blepharoplasty incision in the lower lid. If extra volume is needed the lateral orbital rim and anterior part of the lateral orbital wall may be removed (18.6).

18:5   Decompression of the medial orbital wall and floor

18.5a

Make an incision in the skin 1–2 mm below the lash line and extend it laterally then downwards at the lateral canthus.

18.5b

Deepen the incision to expose the tarsal plate. Dissect down between the orbicularis muscle anteriorly and the tarsal plate and septum posteriorly as far as the orbital rim. During the dissection fat may prolapse through the septum. If this occurs carefully excise the prolapsed fat without traction (see 10.6c,d) and ensure haemostasis.

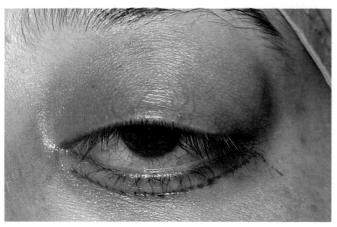

Fig. 18.5a

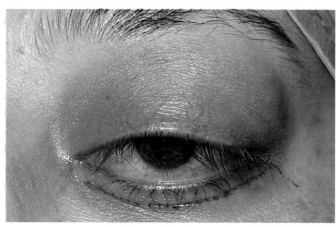

Fig. 18.5b

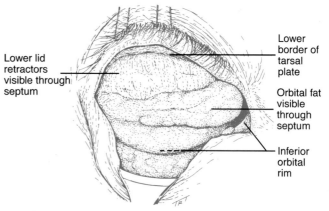

Lower lid retractors visible through septum

Lower border of tarsal plate

Orbital fat visible through septum

Inferior orbital rim

Key diag. 18.5b

Decompression of the medial orbital wall and floor

18.5c

Incise the periosteum along the orbital rim. Using a sharp periosteal elevator raise the periosteum of the rim. With a blunt dissector extend the dissection posteriorly raising the periosteum of the orbital floor and medial wall. The origin of the inferior oblique muscle is often disinserted with the periosteum.

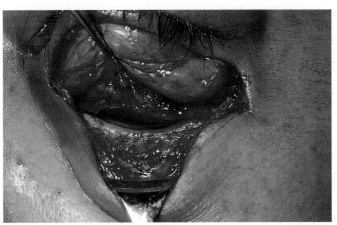

Fig. 18.5c

18.5d

Insert a malleable retractor to displace the globe and soft tissues laterally. Take care to release the pressure of the retractor on the globe at regular intervals.

Using an artery clip perforate the thin bone (arrow) of the orbital floor medial to the infraorbital nerve. Preserve the mucosa of the maxillary antrum if possible but no special action is needed if it is perforated.

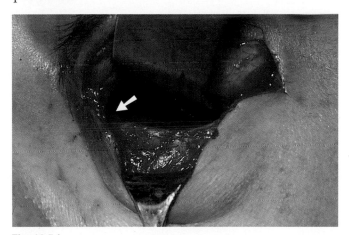

Fig. 18.5d

Technique continues overleaf ➔

18:5 **Decompression of the medial orbital wall and floor** *(Continued)*

18.5e

Using rongeurs carefully remove the medial part of the orbital floor as far posteriorly as the posterior wall of the maxillary antrum. Take care to avoid the infraorbital nerve laterally and the nasolacrimal duct medially. Continue the bone removal up the medial wall as far as the junction with the roof at the fronto-ethmoid suture. The anterior and posterior ethmoid vessels are encountered at this level and they should be preserved. Cauterise them if they are severed. Carefully remove the posterior part of the medial wall in small pieces with an artery clip. Do not go beyond 3 cm posterior to the anterior lacrimal crest – leaving about 1 cm of wall anterior to the optic foramen. Remove all the ethmoid air cells and fine bony septa with an artery clip or sinus forceps.

Incise the periorbita longitudinally in several places to release the orbital fat (arrow).

18.5f

Close the skin incision with a continuous 6/0 monofilament nylon suture as far as the lateral canthus then interrupted sutures laterally. Apply gentle but firm pressure to the closed lids to encourage fat to prolapse into the extra space created. Prescribe an antibiotic such as a cephalosporin for 5 days.

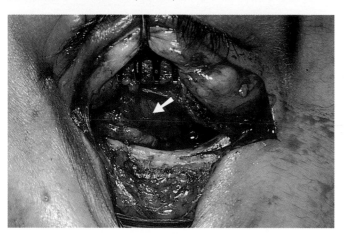

Fig. 18.5e

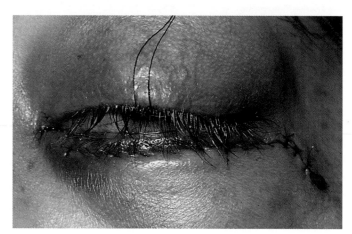

Fig. 18.5f

Decompression of the medial orbital wall and floor

Alternative procedure

In addition to decompression of the orbital floor medial to the infraorbital groove the lateral part of the floor may be decompressed and the infraorbital nerve deroofed. Relatively little extra volume is created by this and the nerve is put at increased risk.

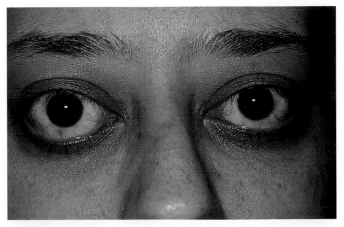

Fig. 18.5 pre

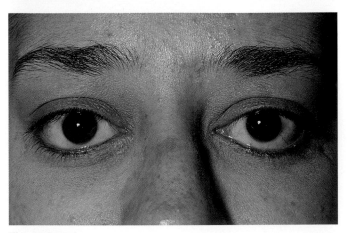

Fig. 18.5 post

Complications and management

Haemorrhage into the maxillary antrum is common if the mucosa has been opened. This resolves spontaneously but some surgeons recommend an antrostomy at the time of the decompression.

Relatively little improvement in the proptosis may result in the early postoperative days. Further improvement may follow a reduction in oedema.

The eye movements may be affected by decompression resulting in diplopia not present preoperatively. Wait for about 6 months before surgical correction.

Extension of the fracture line superiorly into the cribriform plate (with cerebrospinal fluid leakage) or posteriorly into the sphenoid bone around the optic nerve (with variable loss of function in the nerve) are fortunately uncommon. A neurosurgical opinion should be sought if CSF leaks.

18:6 | Decompression of the lateral orbital wall

The lateral orbital wall is formed by the zygomatic bone anteriorly and the greater wing of the sphenoid posteriorly and is at an angle of 45 degrees to the medial wall (see Diag. 1.14). The suture between the zygomatic and sphenoid bones runs almost vertically from the anterior end of the inferior orbital foramen, about one-third of the way back towards the apex of the orbit. Just posterior to this suture the bone of the lateral wall becomes thicker and this warns of the proximity of the middle cranial fossa.

To decompress the lateral wall the lateral orbital rim and anterior part of the wall are removed. The lateral rim, normally replaced in a lateral orbitotomy, may be left out if this improves the decompression. Alternatively it may be wired back but in a more anterior position.

18.6a

Make an S-shaped incision, from immediately below the lateral third of the eyebrow, curving down outside the lateral orbital rim and posteriorly onto the anterior half of the zygomatic arch.

18.6b

Incise the skin and subcutaneous tissues down to the periosteum. Undermine the flaps anteriorly and posteriorly.

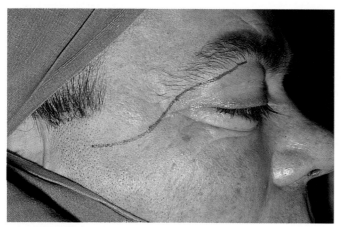

Fig. 18.6a

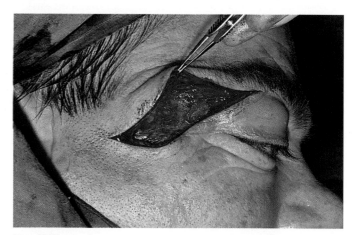

Fig. 18.6b

18.6c

Continue undermining to expose the full extent of the lateral orbital rim, the anterior zygomatic arch and the adjacent temporalis fascia. Place three 4/0 traction sutures in each flap. Incise the periosteum 2mm outside the anterior edge of the lateral orbital rim and along the middle of the zygomatic arch. Carefully reflect the periosteum anteriorly and posteriorly, with a periosteal elevator, to expose the bone of the whole lateral orbital rim.

Continue the anterior reflection of periosteum around the anterior edge of the orbital rim, where the periosteum is firmly attached, into the orbit and elevate the periosteum from the lateral wall.

Continue the posterior reflection of periosteum to the anterior margin of the temporal fossa. Make a relieving incision in the temporalis fascia over the anterior part of the origin of the temporalis muscle from the side of the skull. Dissect the periosteum from the anterior margin of the temporal fossa and continue the dissection into the fossa around the posterior aspect of the frontal process of the zygomatic bone until the lateral orbital wall is exposed.

Mark the positions of the intended bone cuts in the orbital rim – the inferior one just above the zygomatic arch and parallel to it, the superior one just above the zygomatico-frontal suture. Protect the eye with a malleable retractor and drill a hole each side of each mark. The holes are full thickness through the orbital rim and they will allow the bone to be wired back into place if necessary.

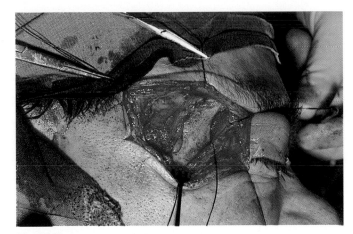

Fig. 18.6c

Technique continues overleaf ➔

18:6 Decompression of the lateral orbital wall *(Continued)*

18.6d

Using an oscillating saw, and with the eye protected, make the lower bone cut first and continue it posteriorly into the lateral orbital wall, parallel to the zygomatic arch for a few millimetres. Make the upper bone cut and continue it posteriorly into the lateral orbital wall in the temporal fossa then inferiorly, parallel to the lateral rim to meet the lower cut. Both the drill bit and the saw blade must be irrigated with saline to prevent overheating.

Remove the lateral rim and orbital wall bone and place it in warm Ringer's solution if it is to be replaced. Using rongeurs remove the remaining thin bone from the posterior part of the lateral orbital wall until thicker bone is encountered.

Identify the lateral rectus muscle within the periorbita. Make several longitudinal incisions in the periorbita above and below the lateral rectus muscle to allow the orbital fat to prolapse.

18.6e

If replacement of the lateral orbital rim causes an obvious increase in proptosis it may be left out.

If it is replaced trim its posterior border of as much thin lateral wall bone as possible and wire it back into position with stainless steel wire. Twist the wire to tighten, cut the ends and turn them medially to prevent erosion through the skin.

Whether or not the lateral rim is replaced close only the anterior periosteum at the orbital rim with interrupted 4/0 catgut. Reattach the anterior origin of the temporalis muscle. Place a vacuum drain in the temporal fossa and out through a stab incision in the skin over the zygomatic arch.

Close the subcutaneous tissues with interrupted 6/0 catgut and the skin with a subcuticular 4/0 monofilament nylon. Remove the drain after 24 hours and the skin suture at 10 days.

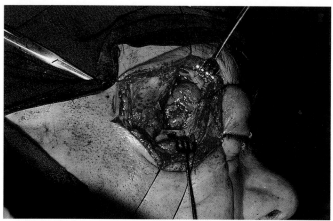

Fig. 18.6d

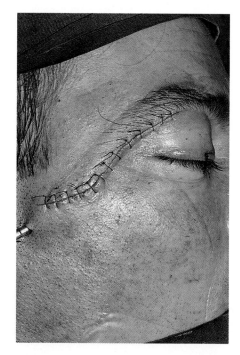

Fig. 18.6e

Temporalis fascia and muscle —

Orbital rim —

— Orbital rim
— Lacrimal gland
— Orbital fat visible through periorbita

Key diag. 18.6d

Decompression of the lateral orbital wall

FURTHER READING

Anderson R L, Nowinski T S: The five flap technique for blepharophimosis. Arch Ophthalmol 107: 448; 1989

Baylis H I et al: The transantral orbital decompression (Ogura technique) as performed by the ophthalmologist. Ophthalmology 87: 1005; 1980

McCord C D: Orbital decompression for Graves' disease; exposure through lateral canthal and inferior fornix incision. Ophthalmology 88: 533; 1981

Mustardé J C: Repair and reconstruction in the orbital region, 3rd edn. Churchill Livingstone, Edinburgh; 1991

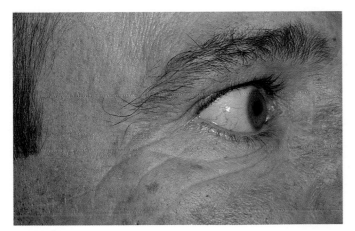

Fig. 18.6 post

Complications and management

Significant haemorrhage into the orbital tissues is uncommon. The orbit is already decompressed so the danger to the optic nerve from the haemorrhage is slight.

Infection is also uncommon and is treated as an orbital cellulitis.

Index